Sheila Mary Taylor was born in Cape Town of Scottish immigrants – Dr James Garden Taylor, psychologist, behavioural scientist and author, and Dora Taylor, novelist, poet, playwright and literary critic. After matriculating at Rustenburg High School for Girls, Sheila studied at the Cape Technical College, and also trained at the University of Cape Town Ballet School, after which she went to the UK to further her career as a dancer. Instead she met and married Colin Belshaw, a mining engineer, and the couple immigrated to Northern Rhodesia (Zambia) where their three sons were born. Sheila took an active part in amateur dramatics and was a keen golfer. When their youngest son developed primary bone cancer, Sheila sat for many hours at his hospital bedside in London, and driven by the drama of his situation she began to write about the incredible battle they fought together.

This true and thought-provoking story, *Fly With a Miracle*, published by Denor Press, was re-published under the title *Count to Ten* by Night Publishing/Taylor Street Books in San Francisco, where until April 2014 Sheila was chief editor. In 2014 Precious Oil Publications published a third edition of *Count to Ten*.

Bardel Publishing has now published a fourth edition of this emotional, action-packed true story.

With one more to go – *Golden Sapphire* – all Sheila's books are now published by Bardel Publishing.

Sheila and Colin spend six months of the year in Cape Town, the other six in Menorca and the UK. She loves music, photography, walking on the beach, and dancing. Her love for ballet never left her and this love has inspired a number of her books.

Also by Sheila Mary Taylor:

Pinpoint

Dance to a Tangled Web

Golden Sapphire

Lari's Castle

Eldorado

Books edited by Sheila Belshaw

Kathie

Don't Tread on My Dreams

Rage of Life

(by Dora Taylor and published posthumously by Penguin)

COUNT TO TEN

- Fly With A Miracle -

Sheila Mary Taylor

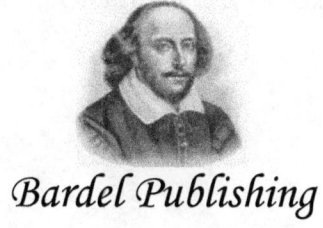

Bardel Publishing

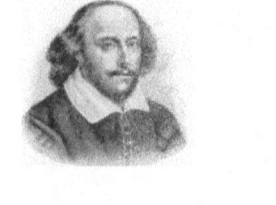

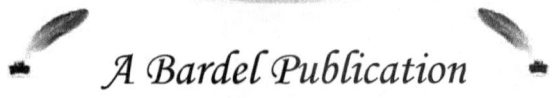
A Bardel Publication

Published by Bardel 2017
© Sheila Mary Taylor 1999, 2011, 2014 & 2016

4th Edition
Count to Ten

First published in 1999 by Denor Press, London
as *Fly With A Miracle* by Sheila Belshaw

2nd Edition published in 2011 by Night Publishing,
as *Count to Ten* by Sheila Mary Taylor
3rd edition published in 2014 by Precious Oil Publications
4th edition published by Bardel Publishing

Permissions

Except for the late Sir Rodney Sweetnam, and the eminent doctors Professor Justin Cobb, Dr Anthony Jellifffe and Dr Gordon Blunn, who kindly gave permission for their real names to be used, as well as the family of Sheila Mary Taylor, the late Dr Philip Rodin and Mrs Jocelyn Rodin, and other close friends, the names of several of the other characters in the book have been changed to protect their identities.

6

experience. The events as they unfold are nothing short of a miracle. Miracle or not, tough and testing times lay ahead for the family." **'Flight path from Hell'** *Sunday Tribune*, **(South Africa)**

"Sheila Belshaw [Sheila Mary Taylor] has written a book about courage that no mother will be able to put down . The book has an immediacy and freshness that makes it compulsive reading." *Cape Argus*, **Cape Town**

"A Story of Hope. Although at times deeply moving, *Fly with a Miracle* is far from depressing. It's a trip that will leave you drained but lifted." **Book of the Week***, Falkirk Herald* **(Scotland)**

Having been a sufferer myself, I found this book more than just a little interesting. The story is about a boy suffering from cancer of the bone, told by his mother. She obviously has deep feelings, and they come across in the story. I suppose 'inspiring' could be the word. It is a good read." **L. Signy, Surrey, England. (5 stars on Amazon.co.uk)**

"What a wonderful story – beautifully told". **Dr Philip Rodin, Consultant Physician.**

In loving memory of Dr Philip Rodin
1931 – 2007

And for my son

Andrew Michael Taylor Belshaw

who never gives up the fight

Foreword

by

Professor Justin P. Cobb Mch FRCS
Chair of Orthopaedics, Imperial College, London

COUNT TO TEN is an amazing story that gives hope to any family going through the terrible experience of cancer as it deals with far more than just the illness. The painful personal details of life are explored in a way that is never less than compelling.

Sheila Mary Taylor has told a story of a family's journey through the horrors of teenage cancer and its aftermath. Andrew marches out the back of the book twice the man he was when he entered it. His astonishing achievements are an inspiration to all.

The author vividly paints a picture of medicine through the 1980s and 90s from a Harley Street experience that nearly ended badly, through the tribulations of the National Health Service with its ups and downs. Her battles to get the best for her son, and the fortunate interventions of friends and hospital staff certainly opened my eyes to the impact the occasional careless word might have on anxious ears.

In this book, the high point for me as a surgeon is the reaction of Andrew and his family to Sir Rodney's initial operation, which I think describes the feelings about amputation and its avoidance more lucidly than ever I could.

This is in part a medical triumph, but in greater part it is a reflection of a vigorous family unit reacting and developing under very great strain and emerging the stronger for being tested like this.

Acknowledgements

There are many people I would like to thank for their invaluable help in the creation of this book. I am grateful to them all, even though I'm unable to mention all their names individually.

The late Dr Philip Rodin and his wonderful wife Jo for suggesting it in the first place after reading the motley collection of notes I had scribbled – and for much, much more.

The late Sir Rodney Sweetnam who explained his orthopaedic wizardry to me, and without whose ground-breaking surgery so many children's lives would not be what they are today.

Professor Justin Cobb for his very generous Foreword and for his technical advice, but above all, for the outstanding ongoing medical advancement he has made to the treatment of osteosarcoma.

Dr Anthony Jelliffe for reading the first draft, and for his wise counselling and encouragement.

Dr Gordon Blunn for his backroom expertise, so often unacknowledged.

Professor Souhami and the staff at The Middlesex Hospital (now sadly defunct), and the London Bone Tumour Clinic, who answered endless questions.

Dr Manasseh Phiri and the late Dr Monica Fisher of Kitwe, Zambia, who both read the first draft and told me to keep going.

Simon Marsh, Andrew's old school friend, for a fresh point of view.

John Holt, best-selling thriller author, for his excellent graphic creation of the 4th edition cover.

My family for their love, patience, support and encouragement.

And in particular, Andrew, for his last minute literary contributions to the book, taken from his diary which I had never seen until just before publication, and whose bravery and fighting spirit are what this book is all about.

'My tale is not for tears

Though sorrow brims the soul;

But rather an exultation

For the spirit of man that takes all

In its compass, to its inmost fibre

Quick and sensible

That dies proudly

Because it knows

That it gave its all to live

Nothing withholding.'

Dora Taylor (1899 – 1976)

'Tristan and Iseult'

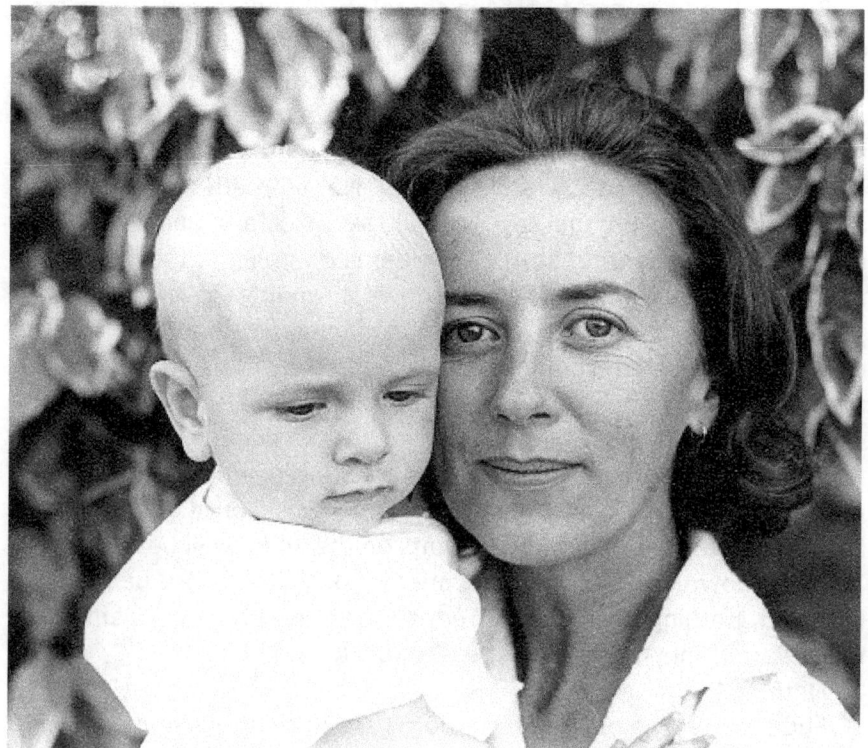

I haven't the faintest idea how the knife got into my hand.

It was a present long ago from a Norwegian friend visiting the Zambian Copperbelt, and I don't remember seeing it around for years. It is one of those huge hunting knives with a short, thick, razor-sharp blade. The handle is bone, roughly carved and far too big really for my small hands.

I look curiously at the knife, and in the moonlight shafting through the open window I see the blade glint. It startles me. I breathe in deeply. The aromas of the African night tantalise my senses with a fragrant cocktail of frangipani, jasmine and gardenia, spiked with wood smoke curling from the myriad fires I see flickering in the bush from Chililabombwe to the nearby Congo border.

Andrew is lying on his bed. It is a warm, sticky October night. He always kicks his bedclothes off, not only in the hot humid season before the rains break but also in the cool July nights of Zambia's

17

tropical winters, so it's not unusual for me to go in and cover him up before I go to bed.

But how odd to see him lying there absolutely naked. There's no sign of his pyjamas and I cannot think what he has done with them.

He is lying quite still. I watch. Waiting for a movement, as I always do. When there is none I feel the first pangs of panic. Then a faint flutter tells me he is breathing after all and I breathe again too.

The night is also still. As still as death. Not a breath stirs the canvas of leaves painted on the vast moonlit sky. Not a sound breaks the rhythm of distant drums, save an eagle-owl do-ooing to the moon, and the muted chorus of frogs in the shadows shrouding the pool.

I look down at Andrew, lying there so still. His body is pale, the curves of the smooth young limbs highlighted by the stark light of the moon.

I move. Stealthily. The moonlight catches the edge of the knife.

I stop. How strange! The blade is pointing downwards as though with a will of its own, appearing thicker as it twists once or twice in my hand. And see how it flashes and glints on the white wall beside me.

I look down again at the pale, pristine skin. Like a rose petal newly bloomed, nothing has ever marred it. I love it with all my being. It is mine. Part of me. Nothing must ever spoil it.

Nothing.

Suddenly, at the edge of my vision, I see again the glint of the knife blade on the wall.

I see the knife blade strike the pristine skin. I see it penetrate the flesh. The flesh is not as soft as it looks. It is firm and resilient. It resists the knife blade.

But now the blade lifts upwards and bright red blood spills from the gash in the flesh. I see the blade come down again. And again. And again. And all I can see now is blood blood blood on the perfect pale skin.

But no longer is it perfect.

I see the heinous knife still in my hand. The heinous, wayward, satanic knife. I open my mouth to scream then hurl the knife deep into the ghostly shadows of the garden. The frogs stop croaking. The crickets stop chirping. The moon looks down and beckons me but I turn my back on it and run.

I must get away. Away from the ruined body. As far as I can. But the knife has drained my energy. My legs are wooden and I can barely

18

move.

I squeeze my eyes closed. I force my legs to move. I push through the thick air to the door. I reach the next room but cannot go further. I collapse into the big brown chair where Andrew and I watch television, cuddled up together like a mother cat and her kitten.

You can't possibly have done it. You love him too much. My voice is strange, strangled and disbelieving.

There is no other sound. Not even a whimper. Only my own feverish breathing as slowly the horror dawns on me that never again will I see that perfection. That beautiful pale skin. Those blue eyes. That golden hair.

That smile.

Why?

I love him. I can't have done it. But there is no-one else here. Who can it have been but me?

It must be a dream. I wish he would cry. Then I would know it is only a dream. But if it is a dream I would be awake by now. You always wake up when ghastly things happen in dreams and nothing could be more ghastly than this.

But I *am* awake. Grossly, grotesquely, gallingly awake . . .

What's that?

A noise. A voice. A bit like laughter.

Laughter?

Yes. There it is again. Like the echo of a laugh, coming from a long way away. A mean, acerbic, caustic, *cackling* laugh. An accusing laugh. Derisive. Mocking.

Scathing . . .

I hear a second voice joining in the laughter. Getting closer. The two voices are getting closer and closer, louder and louder and now there's a third voice and a fourth and a fifth. The voices are all around me now. Hundreds. Laughing loudly. They must be in the next room. The room where I –

Oh no!

At any moment they will come through that door. I cannot face them. I must get away. But how? My legs refuse to move.

I throw my head down on my knees, draw my limbs in like a threatened tortoise, cover my eyes and my ears and my nose to shut out the horror and the laughter and the smell of blood ...

Now the laughter is deafening. How can they laugh at a time like

19

this? I try to scream, to tell them to go away but nothing comes out except my own silent twisted thoughts ...

Guilt. Punishment. Guilt ...

The voices pulse through my body so I know now that they are right here in this room.

Suddenly the laughter stops.

There is an eerie hush. I dare not breathe. What will they do to me? Why don't they get it over with? What are they waiting for? I can't bear it any more.

I feel something touch me. Someone is forcing my head up and someone else is putting ... someone is putting something down across my knees. Something heavy. Something warm. Something clammy, droopy, wet –

Something absolutely still.

I will not look.

Whatever it is I do not want to see it.

Again I hear the voices. Whispers first, growing to soft murmurs. I sense them all around me but I keep my eyes tightly closed.

The voices move away. I force my eyes to open. The moon beams straight in through the window and my eyes are dragged to the heavy warm clammy thing lying limp and unrecognizable across my knees.

I gather it into my arms. This mutilated body. And crush it to my chest. And rock it to and fro as my tears drip on to the once perfect flesh to mingle with the bright red blood. I hold it. This mutilated body. I stroke it and try to coax the life back into it, willing it to be whole again, willing it to breathe, willing it to move, willing it to live and breathe and move and laugh and cry –

But nothing happens, and all I hear is a loud buzzing in my ears.

I close my eyes and press my own wet cheek against that poor blood spattered cheek.

Then suddenly, over and above the buzzing, I hear my own voice and I am shouting:

Live! Live! Live!

Chapter One

October – December 1983

It seemed like a pretty ordinary day.

An ordinary happy-go-lucky day in the middle of Africa. There was no big black cloud darkening the sun. No omen of tragedy.

It was October and the parched bush blistered in the heat. The rains had not broken and the temperature was still rising, though up here on the pinnacle of Kamenza Hill it was just tolerable. (*Ka - men - za*. Say it slowly and you get a feeling of the meaning of the word: *I see a long way*.)

Whipped by a hot dry breeze the pool glistened with the jewels of a thousand suns, enticing me into its delicious depths. I lived either in it or next to it, flopped in my woven grass chair in the shade of the towering African Flame tree with my tea tray and my pile of books scattered next to me on the crooked granite table.

I glanced at my watch. It was almost lunch time. Colin would be home soon. He would be bringing the mail and I wondered if there would be a letter from Andrew.

I gazed across the shimmering bush towards the distant Congo hills. Chililabombwe – *the place of the croaking frogs* in the local language – is the smallest, most northerly mining town on the Zambian Copperbelt, though the richest in copper ore. I was thankful that we lived on top of the only hill for many miles around, for a hot breeze is better than no breeze at all. From down below all you could see was bush. But from up here, if I half closed my eyes, the dusty green of the bush slid silkily into the blue of the sky and I could imagine the shimmering bush was the sea that I missed so much, even though the nearest sea was two thousand miles away.

It was Friday and I was thinking about Andrew.

He was a good communicator and his letters from school arrived promptly once a week. It would be cold in England now. The trees would be bare and it would be raining. He would be cosily wrapped in

21

a thick grey sweater hidden beneath his black academic gown which was the day-time uniform at Bradfield College.

Colin and I missed our sons but this was the price we paid for living in a developing African country. Most good mining jobs are in far-flung foreign countries so we had little option but to live abroad. The local schooling here wasn't suited to the children of expatriates. It was geared more to learning how to make a living from the red earth of Africa. And here there would be no guaranteed employment for our sons so although born in Zambia they had to be educated to live in the outside world in the future. In the end though, the colonial type boarding school in Rhodesia (Zimbabwe), followed by an English Public School resulted in a good balance for our three sons, especially as they came home three times a year to the Zambia they loved.

"It's not doing me any harm," Andrew told me once, even though he hated the English prep school he had been forced to go to when the war in Rhodesia forced the closure of his beloved Whitestone School in Bulawayo. He was only eleven when he'd been catapulted into a completely different environment where the rest of the boys had been since the age of six or seven. They all knew each other, their friendships were forged and Andrew was an alien.

But that was a long time ago. He was eighteen now. He was happy now. He loved Bradfield College. Life was full and exciting even though the school was tucked away deep in the Berkshire countryside. He was a prefect, played cello in the orchestra, shot small bore rifle in the First Eight, swam in the First Team, and played hockey, squash and golf. But most importantly he was a corporal in the Combined Cadet Force. The Air Force section of course, since his dream from the age of eight was to be a pilot in the RAF. I can still see him – that little blond-haired boy, staring up at his bedroom ceiling at the model planes Colin had made for him, hands on his hips as he announced:

"I'm going to be a pilot when I grow up."

A dream that had been intensified when he became an air cadet at the age of fourteen, when flights in Chipmunks at nearby RAF Abingdon were a regular source of inspiration.

I heard a car door slam. A few minutes later Colin was standing at the top of the granite steps leading down to the pool, waving the bundle of mail he brought home every day from the copper mine where he worked as a mining engineer. Quickly I picked up my towel and hurried up the steps to greet him.

22

He tossed the bundle of mail onto the mukwa coffee table that Sikweya Banda polished every day so vigorously that I could see my face in it. I grabbed the familiar airmail letter from the bottom of the pile, reached for the copper letter knife and slit open the flimsy blue sheet.

There were the usual bits of school news, and then … what was this?

A game of hockey … a kick on the shin … pain …

Colin looked up from his *Times of Zambia* as I read from the letter.

"It's not like Andrew to complain of pain," he said.

"I'm sure it's nothing," I mumbled as I finished reading the letter. He was our third son and we were used to the injuries boys of that age received. Besides, we were five thousand miles away and he would be getting the necessary treatment from the school doctor, so we were sure it would get better soon.

Ours was a happy and successful family and things always got better.

How were we to know that this was the beginning of a nightmare? A nightmare I had always thought could only happen to other people.

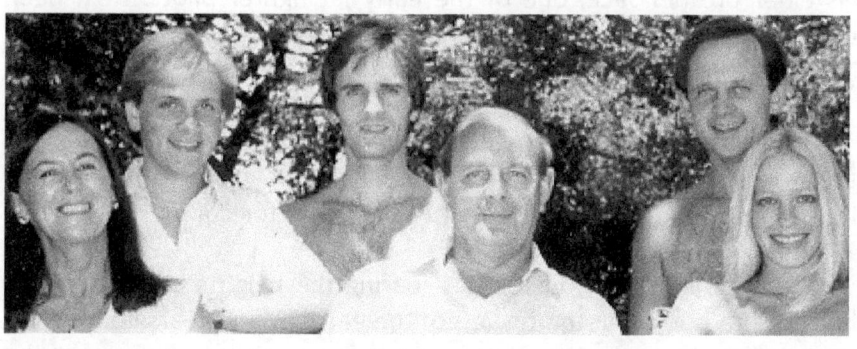

Happy family
Back row: Andrew, Colin jnr, Peter. Front row: Sheila, Colin, Heather

- 0 -

I loved the life in Zambia. Carefree and idyllic, pulsing with the vibrancy of a young country striving for its identity, it offered a challenge to anyone with a sense of adventure. Mine employees lived in spacious modern houses with large gardens boasting the most colourful and

23

fragrant flowering trees and shrubs I have ever seen: flaming flamboyants; scarlet, pink and peach hibiscus; pink and white frangipani; cascades of purple, pink and orange bougainvillaea, and tall graceful jacarandas with their clusters of illusory lilac bells that left carpets of petals beneath their delicately scrolled trunks.

School holidays were a merry-go-round of swimming, riding and golf; bumping through the bush in a Land Rover to visit unspoilt game parks, and sailing on the local dam in our unsinkable old GP-14. The climate was the most perfect in the world and I had servants to do everything.

Yes. It was paradise for me and the children but not always easy for Colin. Sometimes I thought he was too ambitious. Not for himself but for the whole mining industry. The reserves of copper and cobalt were seemingly inexhaustible but it was not a smooth road. Greed and corruption were rife and often I looked at his tired tense face at the end of another long day and thought how much happier he'd have been in a flying career. Not that he didn't love mining, but flying had been his first love. At seventeen he'd been offered a place at the Royal Air Force College, Cranwell, intent upon following in the footsteps of his elder brother Jack, one of the early jet fighter pilots. He'd been poised on the threshold of his promising career when suddenly tragedy had struck.

Jack was killed when his Meteor exploded in mid air.

His grief-stricken father, who had served with the RAF throughout the war, wielded the axe that would splinter Colin's dreams into tiny little pieces. There would be no Air Force career for Colin.

Not over his dead body.

Then, paradoxically, instead of soaring the heights of the heavens he chose to burrow in the bowels of the earth. Many years later he did learn to fly. He worked most of his first love out of his system but the dreams were still there.

And to his youngest son Andrew he imparted those dreams. Dreams that had already begun to come true, when at age seventeen Andrew was chosen to have selection tests at Biggin Hill, and then at the end of the previous term the wonderful news that he was offered a prestigious RAF Flying Scholarship.

I re-read Andrew's letter slowly. Savouring every word as I always did. Remembering the big round uneven writing of his first letters which you knew the teacher had made him write once a week but were none-the-less sweet for this discipline. When he'd gone away to prep school in Rhodesia at the age of six, I was devastated. I had bought my first Poodle then, knowing another child was impossible after the difficult pregnancy I'd had with Andrew.

When we were engaged we had planned four children. Colin, Peter, Andrew and Susan were to be their names. Colin and Peter arrived in quick succession and for a while the family seemed complete. But I'd known all along they would have to go away to school and secretly I began to yearn for another child.

Then one day soon after Peter had joined Colin eight hundred miles away at Whitestone School in Bulawayo, the need became a reality. I was having afternoon tea with Beth, a friend from the amateur dramatic society. Beth was very gregarious and one of her party tricks was to read tea cups.

"You're going to travel a great deal," she said, gazing into my cup, "and – good heavens! I can see three children here."

I laughed, because I'd done nothing to prevent conception all these years yet had not become pregnant again, and also because there was no way she could have known that I desperately wanted another child.

"Let's look at your palm," Beth said. She grasped my hand. After a few moments she confirmed her first forecast.

"There's no doubt about it," she announced gleefully. "You will have *three* children."

And that was it. At that very moment the desire crystallized and the following day I saw the gynaecologist at the Mine Hospital in Chililabombwe.

- 0 -

I went through Andrew's letter once more, trying to read between the lines. I was sure he would be fine. He was so well adjusted and always bounced back quickly. I'd been certain in the beginning that at six years old he was far too young to leave home, but from the very first day he thrived on boarding school. He did reasonably well academically. He was much better at the subjects he enjoyed, like English, and lazy when it came to the ones he didn't like, but always entered enthusiastically into all sporting and social activities.

He would amaze me the way he would go fearlessly towards some new and unknown challenge. At that age he was the most outgoing of

25

our three sons. It was his main asset I think — his special way with people. Even as a little boy he could reach out to people and they would respond to him and want to reach back to him.

I suppose I did tend to spoil him because of the ten year gap between him and his brothers which left him virtually an only child. Otherwise he was absolutely normal. Attractive to the opposite sex too, and lately he always seemed to have a pretty girl at his side.

Thank goodness he had finally got over Emma. Or so it appeared. He had felt bitter at first but no longer bore her any grudges.

"If it breaks up, it breaks up," he said to me a few months after she had ditched him. "You can't make someone love you."

Brave words but at the time I thought he would never get over her. She was lovely. Like a kitten. Petite, tawny-haired, with velvet brown eyes that melted as she smiled. They had seemed so well-suited. They were only seventeen but were truly in love even though they only saw each other during school holidays. I'd been alarmed by the intensity of the relationship. They had even fixed their wedding date. It would never do at this age to make a commitment, I thought, but remembering my mercurial infatuations with boys at that age I had consoled myself that it could not last.

Then came the bombshell. When Emma's father was posted back to Washington the family invited Andrew to go there for his next summer vacation. On his arrival Emma totally rejected him. She had found someone new. With his tender young dreams of everlasting love in ruins he decided after only one week in Washington to book himself on the next flight to Menorca, where his two brothers were on holiday.

I sighed and folded the blue airmail letter. Probably we'd hear no more about his painful leg.

Then suddenly his letters became irregular. Every few days, instead of once a week. He wrote of the pain in his knee and shin every time he played hockey. How he went regularly to see the school doctor, standing in the queue of boys with similar injuries. There would have been no reason to suspect that his painful knee was any different from hundreds of others, so the usual treatment was given: rest for a week and when it was really bad, pain-killing tablets.

But the pain persisted and eventually he was sent for an X-ray. The radiologist saw nothing unusual so nothing was done. The following week he went back to the school doctor. Again nothing was done except to put him off hockey for yet another week.

26

Colin and I didn't even know he had gone for an X-ray because nobody had told us.

- 0 -

In December we were busy moving again. Three hundred miles south to Lusaka, to the head office of the giant copper mining company that was the economic heart of Zambia.

It was our sixteenth move. Our new abode was a large, rambling one-storeyed house in the elegant suburb of Kabulonga. Unlike the Kamenza Hill house with its magnificent views over the bush to the distant borders of the Congo, this house and garden with its kidney-shaped pool and umbrellas of flaming flamboyants was enclosed by a high brick wall topped with shards of broken glass.

I enjoyed the moves. It was a challenge furnishing a new house, creating a new garden, making new friends, playing a new golf course. It diverted my thoughts away from the gap the children left. And from my longing for them to come home.

- 0 -

It was in early December too that I began to grow alarmed at the tone of Andrew's letters. He was finding it more and more difficult to concentrate on his studies because of the pain in his knee. The pain-killing tablets he was forced to take made him drowsy so that sometimes he nodded off in class.

The pressure on A-level students was being stepped up, and to add to Andrew's problems he was being given a bad time by a particularly callous master, who in last term's school report had cruelly written: 'Beach boys don't pass A-levels.' Andrew's golden tan and sun-bleached hair was testimony to his holidays spent at home in Zambia or at our house in Menorca.

The swine. I could have wrung that man's insensitive neck. He gave Andrew no encouragement and at the beginning of December, when due to a delayed train Andrew arrived back half an hour late from a Sunday exeat, this tyrant was waiting to pounce on him. No allowance was made for the painful knee and he was gated for the rest of the term.

Andrew was shattered by the harshness of the punishment, as were

27

all his friends. Not being allowed out also meant he could not even continue with his driving lessons, a restriction which might have proved disastrous later on, had it not been for his dogged determination not to be beaten by this set-back.

As a result of his punishment he was extremely unhappy. Still missing Emma, he phoned us, a rare occurrence since boys were not allowed to make international calls. He told us he wanted to die. And we said reassuringly from five thousand miles away, "Don't be silly, Andrew. You'll get over it."

After each hockey match the doctor put him off for another week and gave him more pain-killers. This went on until the end of the term, with Andrew sometimes visiting the doctor twice a week.

Meanwhile something happened.

Something which appeared quite ordinary at the time but which would have an extraordinary consequence. A wondrous consequence. A consequence totally unforeseen.

I had an operation on both my feet.

Ever since my ballet-dancing days they'd been giving me trouble. To my horror both wounds went badly septic. I could not move any of my toes. I could hardly walk. Shoes were an impossibility because of the swelling. I was offered no physiotherapy and the non-stop pain contributed to my almost total immobility.

I could have killed that surgeon.

- 0 -

I was relieved but apprehensive when Andrew flew home for the Christmas holidays. Hobbling up the stairs to the look-out point at Lusaka airport, I hid my consternation behind my sun glasses, holding my breath as I watched him step from the British Caledonian jet. He walked with hardly a limp and looked surprisingly well and happy. In the car he chatted non-stop, smiling as we bounced along the pot-holed shortcut through the shanty township of Kalingalinga, excited that we were nearly home.

He had not even mentioned his knee.

The rainy season was in full swing now but oblivious of the tropical downpour he was out that very afternoon on the Lusaka golf course. Each morning he went to work with Colin and for five hours studied in a spare office for his A-levels, but in the afternoons and evenings he was caught up in a hectic social life. He played several games of golf that week. Each time he came off the eighteenth green the limp was worse, but as he never complained I did nothing about it.

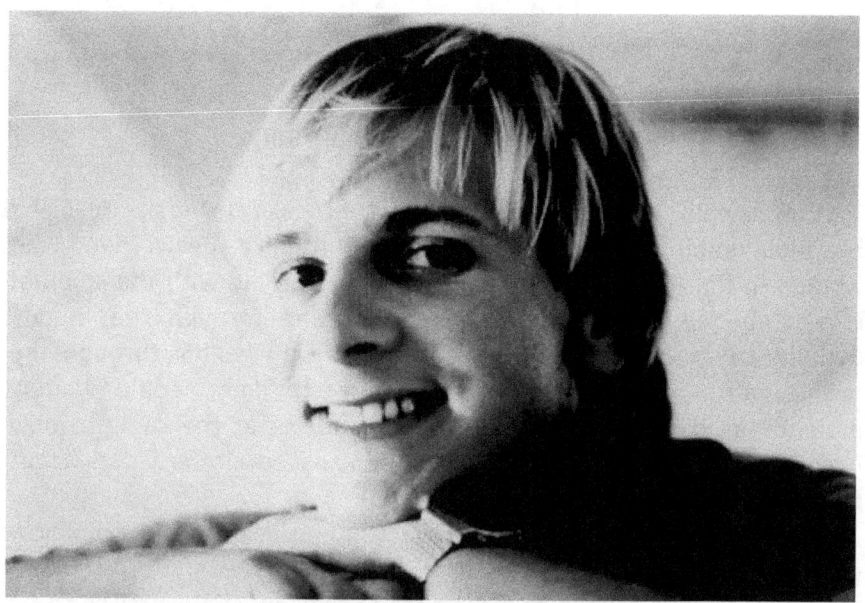

Andrew, age 18, looking so well you would never dream there was anything wrong with him

Then one morning, as I was sitting reading the *Times of Zambia* with my bandaged feet propped up, Sarah, who had been Andrew's devoted nanny since his birth and had followed us to Lusaka, appeared with the tea tray.

"Here's your tea, Madam," she said, her thin face lighting up with a smile.

As I looked up I saw Andrew walking towards me.

Suddenly he collapsed. His leg simply gave way and his body buckled towards it in an effort to ease the pain.

Forgetting my own pain I flew to his side and Sarah and I helped him to a chair.

The pain was mirrored in his crumpled face. Clearly there was something very wrong. Clearly it was time for me to take action.

Chapter Two

December 1983 – February 1984

First we saw an orthopaedic surgeon at the Lusaka University Teaching Hospital, jumping the appointment queue through a special friend who worked in the ICU. We arrived early in the morning with the smell of rain-dampened dust filling the air. Splashing through the muddy puddles to the entrance, we weaved our way guiltily through the milling murmuring crowds: hundreds of shuffling people waiting patiently all day and every day to see a doctor at the capital's only hospital, the steam rising from their rain-soaked clothes, their faces grey with pain and hunger.

After a thorough examination the surgeon said he did not know what it was.

He prescribed daily heat treatment and diagnostic exercises to be conducted by a pleasant, plump physiotherapist, but a week later Andrew could no longer stand the pain of the treatment.

"I'm not going back there, Mum. It's doing me no good whatsoever. And last night when I was out with Cor, my knee gave way again. Just gave way!"

The following day I took him under protest to our local Company GP. An X-ray was taken of his right leg. The GP was baffled.

"It could be a tendon," he said with a worried frown, "but I'd like you to see Dr Scott ..."

I drew in my breath sharply. It was Dr Scott who had recently done Kellers Operation on both my feet to remove my ballet bunions. An operation which in every way had gone horribly wrong. But we had no choice so I said nothing and early next morning Andrew was on his way north to the Copperbelt in the company jet, armed with the latest X-ray.

I sat at home, cursing myself for agreeing to let him go alone. When I picked him up at the airport late that afternoon I couldn't wait to hear the verdict.

30

"Dr Scott reckons it's my cartilage. He offered to operate straight away but I said no."

"Why?" I asked, slowing down at the junction to the Great East Road, half blinded by the setting sun as it sank like an orange ball of fire into the jagged city sky-line.

"I can have it done in England, Mum. It'll be so much easier. And I can have on-the-spot after-care treatment in the school san and still work for my A-levels."

I glanced at him sideways. Andrew was always very persuasive.

He was grinning and I asked him why.

"Mum! You don't really think I'd let that man touch me with a knife, do you? Look at the mess he's made of your feet! No way would I ever let him carve up my knee."

He'd had the guts to say it when I had not. We had no idea at the time what a merciful blessing this was. We had no idea then that any operation, without knowledge of the true nature of the trouble, would have been catastrophic. Further pain would undoubtedly have been attributed to the aftermath of the operation, masking the true cause.

I was meant to have that lousy foot operation. It was meant to go wrong. I was meant to suffer indescribable pain and discomfort. And because I did, Andrew refused to have his cartilage out. He was eighteen and you did not argue with eighteen year-olds with minds of their own.

- O -

But the highlight of that Christmas holiday was Andrew's determination to get his Zambian driving licence.

Seemingly ignoring the pain, he practised every day to make up for the lessons he'd missed in England due to the gating. In no time he was driving my ancient Peugeot far better than I was. He booked a test for early January.

"Just your luck," I said as we arrived at the examining head-quarters in the middle of a blinding tropical downpour that made it difficult to see more than a few yards beyond the windscreen.

First the barrel test. He had practised for hours at a friend's muddy farm off Leopards Hill Road so he had no qualms. Gritting his teeth against the pain he started to reverse the old lumbering Peugeot between the narrow rows of oil drums. There was no power-steering.

31

The rain was still coming down in sheets. He was almost through, but nudged the final barrel.

That was it. He had failed.

He booked a test for the following day but this time he was clever. Since the gap between the barrels remained the same regardless of the size of the car, he borrowed a much smaller car from a friend's mother and had a clear round. A drive through Lusaka's chaotic pot-holed streets completed the test and with his coveted licence he flew happily back to the UK.

Hiding my tears behind my sun glasses I watched his plane soar into the star encrusted sky. As we walked to the car I held Colin's hand.

"He never gives up, does he?"

Colin smiled, then reminded me of a much smaller and younger Andrew, who one morning when he'd become fed up with seeing his equally small friend riding a small bicycle, had announced at breakfast, "I'm going to ride Peter's bike today!" All day he had struggled. His brother's bicycle was miles too big for him. He fell off so many times that I lost count and I couldn't bear to watch any longer. At nightfall he dragged his bruised and battered body into the house. With a huge grin on his face, his big blue eyes sparkling with happiness, he said, "I've done it, Mummy."

Back at school and now free of the gating, he had one more driving lesson and a week later he got his UK licence too.

Even with the painful knee these two achievements were not remarkable, but later, when he could scarcely walk, their enormous importance would be recognised.

- 0 -

January 1984 was the start of the penultimate term of Andrew's school career. There was a great deal of work to do for his A-level exams in July. He needed to be fit to do it but he was anything but fit.

The routine resumed. Hockey. Knock on leg. Doctor. Pain-killers. They made him drowsy, and falling asleep during the day did not help his studying nor endear him to the masters. An entry in his diary in mid January reads:

Managed to struggle through the game against Marlborough today. We lost 1 − 0. My knee gave way

32

again. I wish I knew what it is but then none of the doctors know either.

Certain now that something was very wrong he asked the school doctor to send him for another X-ray. If indeed it was a cartilage problem he felt he should no longer delay having the operation suggested by the surgeon in Zambia.

This time the radiologist did see something.

He saw a distinct pattern of mottling.

A disturbance at the top of the tibia.

Just below the knee.

The X-ray taken in November last year and this new one were compared. A change had occurred in the bone. Andrew was lucky that at last someone had their eyes open.

Alarm bells were rung but Colin and I were not told anything.

- 0 -

One of my greatest passions is ice-skating. Watching it, that is, since beyond the daily lessons I had in Austria for two glorious weeks when my father took me with him to Innsbruck University, I'd had no opportunity to skate. I wanted to skate even more than I wanted to dance but Cape Town had no ice rink when I was growing up, so I had to be content to roller skate.

Colin and I had booked to go to Sarajevo to watch the 1984 Winter Olympics, but once more my lousy foot operation dramatically changed the course of events: I was unable to get proper shoes on my feet, let alone snow boots, so at the last minute we reluctantly abandoned the trip to Yugoslavia and flew to England instead.

Arriving in London the following morning after a sleepless ten hour flight on Zambia Airways, I revelled in the deliciously crisp, cold air. It was a wonderful contrast to the heat of Zambia and so exhilarating to feel your cheeks tingle in the icy wind.

We flew on to Manchester, to our cosy little pied-à-terre near the university where our second son Peter lived while he was studying Law. Oblivious of the bare trees waving wildly in the biting east wind that whistled round the flat, and the constant roar of traffic thundering its way to the city, I sat for one whole week with my feet up and my eyes glued adoringly to the television screen. Not the same as being in

33

the ice stadium at Sarajevo, but a good second best. In Zambia we would have seen nothing.

That weekend Andrew flew up to Manchester for half-term. Peter played hockey every Saturday and had managed to get Andrew a game with his team. He'd forgotten his stick so Colin took him to town to buy a new one.

I looked at him with dismay. "You're not going to play, are you, Andrew?"

"Don't fuss, Mum. My knee will be fine."

He came home limping and laughing at the ridiculous uselessness of his leg.

"Plenty of good peg legs around," Colin said jokingly.

It was Andrew's last game of hockey.

Next day he wrote in his diary:

> I wish I hadn't played hockey yesterday. My knee is now very painful. I couldn't even go out with Mum and Dad today.

The entry the following day:

> Woke up in absolute agony again. Hardly slept a wink, as usual.

And the next day:

> After yet another sleepless and painful night, I flew back to London.

And back at school:

> Had to go to the san today and get some pain-killers after not sleeping again. I wish this blasted knee would clear up.

I only read his diary years later, so I had no idea then how bad the pain was.

And when we had said goodbye to him at Manchester Airport he remarked, casually. "Oh, I almost forgot to tell you. I'm going to have a bone scan on the fifth of March."

I almost stopped breathing. My mind groped but nothing tangible reached out to tell me this was anything I should worry about. Yet for a few seconds I was aware that something dreadful was about to happen.

I always try to think positively, so I dismissed these thoughts instantly. Andrew's face told me nothing. Nor did his tone of voice suggest he was anxious or afraid. I reckon he thought it was just routine. I think Colin did too. And I kidded myself that it was.

We were going to our villa in Menorca for ten days and I put a note in my mental diary that I'd be back in England by the fifth of March, and then thought nothing more about it. I knew nothing about scans or why people had them. In those days no-one in our circle of friends had ever had one, yet there must have been some tiny obscure wisp of information that tried to push its way out to warn me.

Human beings have a clever mechanism for overcoming threatening thoughts. If you banish them from the mind for long enough they will often disappear forever. This is what I subconsciously did with the bone scan and Colin and I didn't even discuss it.

The day before we flew to Menorca we telephoned Andrew at school. He said there was no change and clearly he had no idea that anything really serious might be wrong. He only knew he had a painful leg and that something had to be done to put it right.

We had no idea either. We hadn't been told about the second X-ray in February, nor that a bone scan had been arranged. The school had been totally silent about what was going on.

Why?

Months later it became clear that they had all been very worried indeed. They'd had their suspicions but these were not communicated to us because they were trying to protect us from unnecessary worry. (And only now are GPs being warned to refer to a specialist if a teenager has a persistent ailment because of the vital necessity for early diagnosis.) The school had full in loco parentis charge of the children in their care and were experts at their job. If they were to spread unnecessary panic about every injury they had to deal with there would be chaos.

I agreed with this in theory, yet in hindsight it is clear that a word in the parents' ear about their worry would have shifted the responsibility. Parents should be allowed to make a fuss and insist on immediate action. This finally happened but only a month later. A month that in Andrew's case might have made a very big difference.

When Colin and I set off for Menorca we had no idea that on our return to London our lives would never again be the same.

- 0 -

Menorca's winters can be miserably cold, wet and windy, but it was bliss to be in our villa on the hill with its panoramic views of the sea and the lake and the hills rolling into the distance like miniature Himalayas.

Sitting in two deliciously comfortable reclining chairs in front of the French window overlooking the lake and the sea, we were quite happy just to read. When you got tired of your book you could gaze out at this jewel of a view that was so different from Africa.

Those ten idyllic days were the lull before the storm.

Chapter Three

March 1984

The tramontana woke us early in the morning as it shrieked through the wooden window frames and lashed the wild olive trees surrounding the villa. Not expecting to return until late summer, we closed the shutters, locked the doors, then drove through the hills to Mahon Airport just as the sun struggled through the bank of steel-grey clouds racing along the horizon.

The plan was for Colin to fly straight on to Lusaka while I indulged in a week's feast of ballet and theatre in London. I hate to think what would have happened if I had not been there that week; if I had been in Sarajevo watching the Winter Olympics. But because of my feet I was there. I was able to get things moving. And I was able to phone Philip and Jo.

Philip and Jo Rodin. Who changed the course of Andrew's fate.

- 0 -

My sister Doreen met us at Heathrow. I was to spend the weekend with her and Michael at Pipers Croft before going to stay with their daughter Jenny in London for my week of culture.

Also there to meet us were Dave and Peggy, friends from Menorca. Without their quiet support in the coming weeks I would not have coped.

After a quick coffee together in the restaurant, Colin flew by helicopter to Gatwick to board his flight to Lusaka. As I kissed him goodbye I whispered, "See you in a week, darling," never guessing what lay ahead.

Next morning I set off early to pick Andrew up from school and bring him back to Pipers Croft for the family Sunday lunch. On the way back we stopped off nostalgically at the village pub where my father used to take us before he lost his legs from arteriosclerosis. Where his

37

Scottish jokes used to have the whole pub in stitches. Jokes he always insisted on telling even though he had only once been back to Scotland when Aberdeen University conferred upon him the honorary degree of Doctor of Science.

That evening, just before we drove back to Bradfield College, Doreen asked what it was we were planning to do the next day. When I told her, she frowned.

"Why a bone scan?" she asked.

Everyone turned and looked at me. Waiting for my answer.

I glanced at Andrew, seeking his help. His face was non-committal. Neither of us had mentioned it today and suddenly a cold gust of doubt blew me momentarily off balance.

Spots danced before my eyes. I did not know how to answer her and for the first time, because I actually had to put it into words, I began to formulate in my mind the reality of the situation. Something serious must be wrong but I hadn't a clue what it could be.

"To ... er ... well, I don't know, really." I cleared my throat. "To find out if there's anything unusual wrong. I suppose," I added when they all looked at me blankly

I fiddled with the car keys, turning away to hide the sudden cognisance that leapt into my mind.

"Oh!" Doreen replied, equally awkwardly, and gave me a funny look.

- 0 -

Andrew was waiting outside when I arrived at his House next day. Rushing to the car in a gait that was more a hop than a run, his face twisting in pain, he asked if his three best friends could join us at The Bull, the nearby country pub we were going to for lunch before his appointment at the hospital.

The atmosphere was happy and relaxed, and as we tucked into the enormous ploughman's lunch it was clear that Simon, Stuart and James had no idea that their mate was so near to being snatched prematurely and permanently out of school.

- 0 -

The hospital was a conglomeration of large, old, overheated buildings,

38

connected by a maze of passages and tunnels, and it took us about fifteen minutes to find the Isotope X-ray department.

First they X-rayed his chest. A bit strange, I thought, when it was his knee that was painful. Then, as Andrew clenched his jaw, they injected him with a blue fluid.

"Come back in two hours' time," said the smiling nurse. "By then the fluids will have reached the tissues to be scanned."

On the way out, faint from the injection and the sauna-like heat of the X-ray department, Andrew nearly passed out but was soon revived by a kind nurse who took him outside into the cool air and kept his head down until he recovered.

It was a very long two hours. We tried shopping, then settled for a tea-room. Andrew was restless and I asked him how he felt.

He shrugged. "I'm fine now, Mum. I'm not bothered, really. I'm just glad something is going to be done at last. Though I hope nobody is going to stick any more needles into me."

"Is the pain really bad now?" I asked. He had never really told me.

Biting his bottom lip, he nodded. "Well, it comes and goes, Mum. To begin with it was just a feeling of discomfort. Then it became a dull ache. Then short sharp excruciating stabbing pains followed by ache. Then continuous unbearable ache with stabs like knives. Getting worse each time. Bad enough to stop me sleeping."

I was aghast. "Why didn't you tell me this before?"

"You never asked me."

- 0 -

Once we were back at the hospital the scan was quickly done. While Andrew got dressed I sat sweltering in the green and cream waiting room, wondering what on earth was going to happen. What if he had to have an operation? I would have to delay my return to Zambia. Flights were always full for months ahead so I would have to book soon. I would have to know immediately what the results of the scan were.

Boldly I walked up to the reception desk.

I coughed to attract the girl's attention. "Could I please be told the results as soon as possible," I asked.

She looked at me as if I were mad. "You will be told the results in due course and in the usual manner," she said politely but firmly.

39

I stared at her, wondering what I had done wrong. Timidly I protested and she made a half-hearted attempt to contact the radiologist.

"I can't find him," she said, then repeated that I would get the results in due course.

I learned much later that it is not necessary to accept the impersonal treatment that is so often thoughtlessly handed out by seemingly uncaring people in positions of petty authority. It was my fault. I should have insisted. I should have explained my dilemma, but I didn't know then that if you really are worried and want to have something attended to straight away, there is always someone in a big hospital who will help you. In the beginning I did not know this. I didn't want to be pushy or cause a fuss, and I meekly and stupidly accepted that I would have to wait.

The next few days were torture. Someone could have taken a quick look at that scan, I told myself. Someone could have informed me of the result. But I didn't know then how to ask, so I had to suffer the intolerable torment of waiting.

I delivered Andrew back to school, gave him a kiss and a hug and promised to phone him every day. I drove back to Pipers Croft along the M4, dazed and disorientated, going slower and slower, dazzled by the oncoming lights which first grew brighter, then larger, then started going with me instead of against me.

- 0 -

For my treat week of ballet and theatre I stayed with my niece Jenny Muskett in Highgate. Jenny is a warm, generous person as well as being a talented, Emmy prize-winning composer of music for films, and always makes me feel at home. She and her husband, Michael Rosenberg, who produced award-winning wild-life films, often took Andrew out at weekends, and there was a special bond between them.

Before leaving the house for the CATS matinée, I tried in vain to contact the school doctor. Finally I reached the Sister at the school sanatorium and asked her to please hurry the doctor up and get him to tell me what was going on.

"The doctor has a very busy schedule," she explained. "He won't get a report about the scan until Wednesday or Thursday and then he'll have to study it before he could talk to you."

In other words – they would call me.

I was on the point of swearing at her but slammed down the phone instead. I know it was rude. She hadn't done a single thing wrong but by this time I was beginning to have an inkling of what bone scans were all about. How could they be so unfeeling about something that so critically affected my son's health when it would have been so easy to comment on it straight away?

- 0 -

I had been dying to see *CATS* for ages. I was crazy about all kinds of dancing and had done modern dance myself, as well as ballet. I sat next to a wildly enthusiastic young dancer from New Zealand who jumped up and down and soon had me jumping up and down with him and at the end we stood and shouted our heads off in appreciation.

For two and a half hours I had almost forgotten about Andrew.

Dave and Peggy were waiting for me outside the theatre and took me out for dinner. They kept in touch every day. They didn't ask questions because they knew there were no answers, but they were there. That was the important thing.

- 0 -

The early morning sounds on Highgate Hill woke me with their unfamiliarity. It was still dark but I could swear that beyond the swish of traffic and the rustle of leaves I could hear a nightingale sing. It was probably my imagination but already my mind was deranged by the thought of another day of agonising waiting.

The morning dragged on. I phoned the Sister. She gave me the same story as yesterday but this time I managed to keep my temper.

Jenny spoiled me with cups of Rooibos tea, slices of Marmite toast and my favourite Mozart concertos. She drove me to Brent Cross to do my 'home-on-leave' shopping under one incredible roof instead of trudging up and down Oxford Street. I spent a lot of money. I even laughed. But through the web of distraction crept the relentless tendrils of doubt.

What was wrong with Andrew?

Much Ado About Nothing with Derek Jacobi at the Barbican was my next treat. London Contemporary Dance that evening. Both terrific,

41

but the enjoyment was blotted out by the fear that was stealing like a tapeworm into every crevice of my being.

In the intervals I rushed to the phone. I asked Andrew how he was. "Fine," he said cheerfully, as always.

That night I lay in bed. Eyes wide open. Every minute an hour.

Thursday dawned with the now familiar Highgate nightingale. Even his hauntingly beautiful song failed to distract my one-tracked thoughts.

I sat around all morning, doing nothing. I glared at the phone. I poured another cup of tea. I stared at the cup. I talked to myself:

"If they haven't phoned by the time this cup is empty I will bloody well phone the Sister again. Whether she likes it or not."

I took a sip. The phone rang. I grabbed it before its second ring.

It was the school doctor.

I held my breath.

"The radiologist has reported a hot spot ..."

A hot spot?

What is that?

"... which must be investigated. We must treat this seriously so I have made an appointment for Andrew to see an orthopaedic surgeon tomorrow afternoon at two-thirty."

I wanted to scream but I had to be calm.

I phoned Andrew straight away and though he said he was pleased, in his voice I detected a frisson of fear.

"Thank goodness, Mum," he said. "I can't put up with this pain much longer."

I did not mention the 'hot spot'. Like me he would not understand it and I didn't want to upset him. We would soon find out, I was sure.

I sleepwalked by tube to Covent Garden and picked up my ticket at the Opera House. It was still too early for the ballet so I wandered aimlessly around the quaint touristy shops. At one corner a couple of musicians were playing, coins tinkling into an upturned hat. At another a troupe of acrobats were hair-pinning their bodies into inhuman shapes. Fascinating stuff, but nothing lifted my spirits.

The ballet was exquisite, the Opera House as rich and ornate and exciting to be in as always, but I was unable to enjoy it. In the interval I queued for the phone.

"How are you, Andrew?"

"Fine."

"You don't sound fine. What's wrong?"

"Nothing, Mum. Just frustrated. Why can't these doctors tell me why I have this pain."

"They will soon, I'm sure. I'll pick you up at lunch time tomorrow. I love you."

"I love you too, Mum."

- 0 -

Deep in the Berkshire woodlands our lunch at The Bull is somewhat more subdued today than last time, both of us afraid to voice the questions lurking in our hearts.

We arrive at the clinic at two-thirty. The secretary ushers us in and we sit down opposite the doctor. Across the wide expanse of his polished desk his hooded eyes peer at us from beneath a brow wrinkled like the ridges on a wind-swept beach.

Clutched in his hand is a large brown envelope.

I'm amazed when he does not examine Andrew's leg. He doesn't even look at it. He asks all the usual questions but makes no comment on the answers. Just nods.

He opens the large brown envelope. He puts the first bone-scan on the illuminated frame on the wall and invites Andrew and me to come and look at it.

One glance is enough.

The scan is made up of a sea of little black dots. My eyes are dragged to an area just below the knee. To the site of Andrew's pain. Where an extra thick, dark mass of black dots jumps off the screen.

The hot spot?

I catch Andrew's eye.

I see the first signs of unease.

He whispers in my ear. "Jesus! What the hell is *that*?"

In a single moment all the thoughts lying submerged in my subconscious surge like a tidal wave to the surface of my mind, engulfing me with feelings of bewilderment, doubt and disbelief.

And a slow sinking sliding feeling of fear.

I hold my breath as one by one we examine the X-rays. On the one taken in February, you can see speckles on the tibia. If you screw up your eyes you can even see them very slightly on the first one taken way back in November.

43

So why was nothing done sooner?

My pulse beats wildly. The doctor strokes the stubble on his chin. Something is very wrong and I wait for him to speak.

"The scans of the knee and tibia indicate that there is a hot spot at the top of the tibia in the right leg."

"Hot spot? Why?" Andrew says.

"We don't know," the doctor says. "On the other hand, the scan of the whole body tells us that it is only the tibia that is affected." He pauses, but gives no indication of the implication of this. It means nothing to me and I can tell by the blank look on Andrew's face that it means nothing to him either.

"The chest X-ray which was done on the same day as the bone scans, is clear." he says.

He carries on. "I will do a bone biopsy to see what this hot spot is. This will entail removing a piece of bone from the area and having it examined by pathologists to ascertain the reason for the abnormality."

What abnormality? I wonder. I sob inwardly. Oh no! What is happening to my son?

He asks us to sit down again.

We sit down.

He takes a deep breath. He is obviously having a bad time thinking what to say next.

At last he speaks. This time he looks straight at Andrew.

"I think it could be Paget's disease."

Andrew and I look at each other. We have never heard of Paget's disease.

But I have to know. "Please could you describe to us what this Paget's disease is."

The voice drones on, as though from another world. And he doesn't mince his words. "Paget's disease frequently affects the tibia, but the spine, skull and collar bone could also be affected."

Spine?

Skull?

Collar bone?

"How?" I croak. I look at him with fire in my eyes.

He pauses again, then takes a deep breath. He understands that I have to know everything.

"The bones become enlarged. Misshapen. The legs can become bent and the skull ... the skull becomes bigger. The spine may become curved ..."

Whose legs? Whose skull? Whose spine? What on earth is this man saying? Surely he must be talking about someone else. He can't possibly be talking about my son. This handsome, vital young man sitting next to me. This vibrant, flawlessly formed young man. This strong athletic picture of perfection.

What can he be thinking about?

He is making a jolly good job of plunging us right into the middle of a nightmare. That's what he is thinking about.

And I think he is crazy.

"But as far as we can see at the moment, it is only his right tibia that is affected."

He carries on talking as though he has just told us that Andrew has tonsillitis. "Because Andrew is covered by the school BUPA system I will perform a biopsy as soon as possible, *if* there's a bed available in the private hospital where I work. Or I can do it under the NHS. *If* they have a bed."

Now I am very calm. But I am like an arrow quivering in the bow ready to fly. After all the delays of the preceding weeks and months I want everything to be done now. Immediately. There will be no more stalling. No more waiting. Oh no!

Andrew's expression tells me that he hasn't really taken in the doctor's horrific words.

"Mum," he says. "I'll have the biopsy after our House First Eleven hockey final. I can't possibly let them down." He is a loyal member of his House hockey team, although he hasn't played since the game in Manchester with Peter.

He is soon over-ruled, and apart from that hiccup he is amazingly calm.

The doctor ushers us out. The other patients glower at us and I realise that we have been in the consulting room for almost an hour, though it feels as though time has stood still.

The secretary drops everything to search for a bed for Andrew.

But not one is available.

The first one will be in eleven days' time.

Eleven days!

We cannot wait eleven days.

I pace around the waiting room like a chicken with its head chopped off. The secretary takes us back to the doctor and I suggest we try to get a bed in a London hospital.

"I'm sorry," he says, "but I can't possibly treat Andrew at such a distance from my normal practice."

Right now I don't much care about medical etiquette so I blurt out: "Then do you mind if I take him to see somebody else. In London? Somebody who could perform the biopsy immediately?"

To my surprise he readily agrees, then instructs his secretary to give us the folder with all the X-rays, scans, reports and letters. All except one. First he carefully extracts one sheet of paper and whips it away. Not for my enquiring eyes? I wonder why.

The kind secretary sees us to the door. She takes my hand and squeezes it.

"Good luck," she says.

She smiles a sad smile at Andrew, and then we are outside.

A cold March wind blows across our faces. We stand with our backs close to the door. We button up our coats. I put my arm around Andrew. He hugs me back.

We are all alone and I am frightened. I feel a heavy weight bearing down on me, buckling my knees and crushing my head down into my shoulders.

The world stands still.

Somehow I must get him to another doctor quickly, but right now there is not one single soul out there who is going to do anything about it. Nobody.

Except me.

After the moment of stillness we run to the car. Andrew winces with the pain. It is now four-thirty on a Friday afternoon and we must hurry in order to get things moving before the weekend.

We arrive back at Hillside House. I make a quick phone call from Andrew's housemaster's study to a nursing friend and secure the name of Mr Cedric Adanar, an orthopaedic surgeon in Harley Street.

Andrew goes off to a lesson. How can he act so normally with all this going on? I can only think that nothing has really sunk in.

Paget's disease?

Oh, please, no!

I dial Mr Adanar's number. His secretary is most understanding. She says she will speak to Mr Adanar as soon as he is free, and call me back.

I quickly phone Colin in Zambia. I leave out the Paget's disease bit

46

but he is shocked to hear that Andrew must have a biopsy. I long to comfort him but I don't have time to talk. I blow a kiss down the phone and ring off.

I try to settle down. I walk round and round the room. A million thoughts zigzag through my head. It is nearly six o'clock. If nothing is fixed up soon it will mean waiting the whole weekend, since most consultants disappear on Friday afternoons and only re-appear again on Monday mornings. *Please, let Mr Adanar be able to see Andrew soon. Let him have a bed available in a hospital. Any hospital.*

Please, telephone – ring!

It rings shrilly and I jump as though a bomb has gone off. I tear across the room to pick it up. I glance at my watch and see that I have only waited fifteen minutes though it has seemed like an hour.

Miraculously Mr Adanar's secretary has arranged everything. He will see Andrew at ten-thirty on Monday morning in his rooms. Andrew will be admitted to a private hospital at one-thirty and Mr Adanar will do the bone biopsy at four-thirty.

My heart sings.

We are no longer alone.

When Andrew comes back from his lesson he is a bit fed-up at having to miss the House hockey finals.

He sighs. "Oh, well, I don't suppose with this leg I'd have been much use to the team. Anyway, I can't bear to have the pain go on any longer."

He holds both my hands. "Mum. What's wrong with me?"

He looks at me with those big trusting blue eyes and my heart cries for him.

"Have I got Paget's disease?"

"I don't know, darling, but we'll soon find out." I kiss him goodnight. "Sleep well, my love."

I drive into the darkness of the night and shiver as the chilling fear of the unknown creeps slowly up my spine.

Chapter Four

This was Andrew's last normal weekend at school, though no-one could have known it at the time.

Peter phoned to say he was coming down from Manchester and I knew Andrew would be thrilled to see him. Because of the eleven and nine year gap, Colin and Peter had been more like fathers than brothers to him, and when he was much younger we would tease him about needing three fathers to keep him in order.

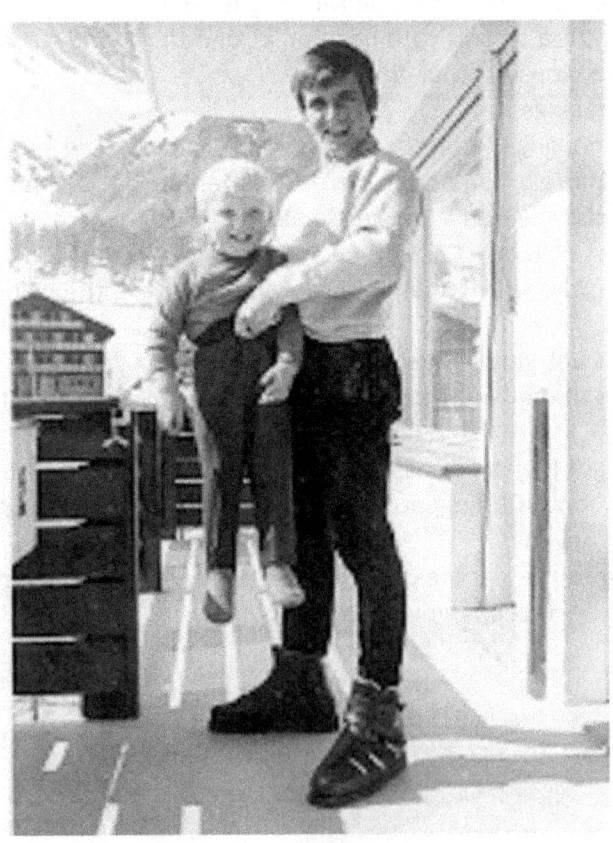

We picked Andrew up at school and took him to a picturesque country pub with a thatched roof and a flickering log fire. In our subdued mood we felt out of place amongst the red-faced Berkshire farmers and their elegantly dressed wives, all speaking at the tops of their voices, drowning our silent thoughts. After our meal we called in at The Bull. This was more relaxing. With no ostentation, everyone joined in the fun and it was good to see Andrew laugh.

Peter and I got back to Pipers Croft around midnight, confident that although it had been difficult to keep entirely off the subject of his knee, we had cheered Andrew up a little. We talked for hours but when finally I got into bed sleep was impossible.

Peter left after lunch on Sunday. He stood at the car and held my hands. "Don't worry, Mum," he said gently. "I'm not far away. If you need me I'll be here."

I stood watching the car drive away until I could no longer see it, then Jenny took me back to Highgate to stay with her while Andrew was in hospital in London.

After unpacking I went for a long walk in Highgate Park and tried to make sense of my mixed-up emotions. Oh, how I missed Colin. He was the only one I could tell my innermost thoughts to but he was five thousand miles away and the phone lines were pathetically useless.

It was a bright afternoon but bitingly cold. I pulled my beret well down over my ears and turned up the collar of my coat. The wind made my eyes water and blew billowing grey clouds across the pale sky as it whistled through the bare branches of the trees and swept down over the city which sprawled before me as far as I could see.

I had never realised before just how far the bond of motherhood could stretch, how acutely I could feel; how closely I could identify with my son as though it were my own fate exposed to the surgeon's scalpel. As I breathed in the bracing air on those windswept paths around the ponds, I remembered as though it were yesterday how thrilled I had been when I knew I was pregnant again, only one month following the small operation I had to have after Beth had read my tea-cup and my palm.

I had been so excited. It was as though I was expecting my first child.

"But the other two are off your hands. Why start all over again?"

49

my friends asked in dismay.

"This one will be special," I told them with a smile.

Others, thankful not to be in my shoes, gave me snide sideways glances as if to say, "Huh! What a stupid mistake at her age! Won't do her golf handicap any good."

I ran up the hill, smiling to myself as I recalled for the first time in eighteen years the very moment of Andrew's birth, amazed at how vividly I could relive the actual moment of him becoming a person. Feeling the slippery aliveness slide between my legs and touch my thighs. Hearing his cry. Seeing his perfect little body and his perfect little head, round and smooth as though he had been delivered by Caesarean section. Holding him close to me. Even after the gruelling thirty-six hours of labour I had been overwhelmed by the intense feeling of wonderment, and tears had flowed freely down my cheeks.

That evening Jenny picked Andrew up from Highgate tube station after his lunch date at his friend Emily's house. Apprehensive about tomorrow's biopsy, he was quiet and solemn, quite unlike the usual talkative Andrew who bubbled over with laughter and fun and infected everyone else with his joie de vivre.

- 0 -

Mr Adanar's petite smiling secretary welcomed us to his Harley Street rooms, as charming as she had been efficient on the phone on Friday afternoon.

Mr Adanar was most concerned about Andrew. He was a tall, slim man, with a shock of prematurely grey hair and soft grey-blue eyes that looked directly at you and made you feel he had all the time in the world for Andrew, and only Andrew.

First he explained that very often sportsmen who have repeated knocks on the same part of a bone develop a condition known as stress-fracture, and this shows up on a bone scan as a hot spot.

There was the word again. Hot Spot. I wondered how soon I would hear the words Paget's disease.

He divided his gaze equally between Andrew and me. Then he said, slowly, "But there is also a possibility that it might be a tumour."

Tumour?

I had kept that word hidden away in the shadows of my mind, but now, for the first time, it had been uttered. I saw it painted in giant red

50

letters across the wall behind Mr Adanar's head, blotting out Hot Spot and Paget's disease.

TUMOUR

Quickly Mr Adanar re-assured us, his buoyant tone adding a hint of hope to his words. "However, I feel sure it is a stress fracture. But if it is a tumour it will probably be benign anyway. The biopsy will provide all the answers."

Direct. To the point. Honest.

I liked his approach, and I saw by the relaxed look on my son's face that Mr Adanar had also succeeded in giving Andrew encouragement and a little bit of hope. Not a word had been said about Paget's disease and I was afraid to ask.

Mr Adanar explained that the blue fluid they had injected into Andrew was called a radio-active isotope. "This zeroes in on parts of a bone which is making new bone. A radiation sensitive camera is then used to produce a picture – different from an X-ray – which shows up the areas where the isotope has concentrated and which are the sites of the bone activity. Increased bone activity – those hot spots – may be due to the repair of a fracture. Or to Paget's disease. Or to a tumour."

I watched Mr Adanar give Andrew a very thorough examination. He even measured his legs. What for, I wondered. To see whether Paget's disease had already made the leg grow longer and thicker? He looked up at me and said:

"The area at the top of the right tibia is very hot to the touch. And very swollen."

Darting back to his desk he leafed through the pile of letters and reports I had brought with me. Then, sensing my curiosity he looked up. He paused, as though carefully weighing up his choice of words, looking from Andrew to me, and back again to Andrew.

"I have never known Paget's disease strike anyone under fifty. Let alone someone of eighteen."

I breathed out. Andrew glanced at me and smiled.

- O -

We were less afraid when we left Mr Adanar. I felt we were in very capable hands and very caring hands and I could see that Andrew had confidence in him.

It was too early to check in at the hospital. Andrew was not allowed to eat anything before his anaesthetic, so to use up the time on our hands we decided to call on Philip Rodin, whose consulting rooms were only a few doors up the road in Harley Street.

Philip and Jo Rodin.

The two people who were responsible for what happened next.

Unfortunately Philip was not in his rooms that day. He was probably at the Royal London Hospital where he worked as a consultant physician. I might never have pursued the contact, but luckily I made a casual phone call to his wife Jo two days later, so in the end the vital link was made.

How touch and go that vital link was!

- O -

From Andrew's diary:

> *Today's the big day.*
> *Mr Adanar had a different story from all the others.*
> *Not cartilage. Not Paget's disease. Perhaps a stress fracture of some kind.*
>
> *That's all I need.*
>
> *First introduction to Nurse Laura and what a laugh she is.*
> *Good looking too. Kind.*
> *Blood test none too entertaining though. The needle.*
> *Pre-med did nothing either so when they came to take me to theatre I was even more frightened.*

- O -

The doors to the private hospital opened automatically, ushering us into a deeply carpeted reception area with the aura of a first class hotel. In his comfortable en-suite room on the fourth floor, Andrew answered questions for the completion of a very large admittance form covering his whole medical history, and mine and Colin's too.

A vivacious looking nurse called Laura then came in to take a blood sample. She jabbed at his arm. Andrew bit his lip. When two more attempts still yielded no blood she discovered the needle had no hole in it, but by the time she succeeded with a new needle Andrew was not very happy, and the whole episode did nothing to help his already deep-seated fear of needles.

Peggy arrived unexpectedly just after Sister had given him the pre-med injection. As well as being neighbours in Menorca we had often met on previous visits to London, and now she and Dave were demonstrating their true friendship. We sat quietly by the window, watching for Andrew to show some signs of going to sleep.

But whatever was in the pre-med appeared to have the opposite effect and he stayed wide awake.

Jo Rodin told me afterwards that with an unknown operation ahead of him he wanted to see what they were going to do to him, and being normal and tough and eighteen he fought against the pre-med effects.

We sat silently. We tried not to look at Andrew but he was not even drowsy. He just kept fighting and my blood ran cold when he told me later that he could even remember the first incision of the knife, though nothing after that. I did not disbelieve him because I had once regained consciousness during a procedure at a hospital in Zambia. My eyes had opened to reveal my legs suspended by ankle straps and I could feel an instrument like a giant plunger dragging out my insides.

At last it was time to go. He had on a shapeless gown and theatre socks, and his leg was shaved from just below the right knee. I held his hand and smiled.

"I'll see you soon, darling. I'll be here when you come back."

I watched them wheel him out. As he disappeared down the passage a now familiar shudder ran down my spine. I turned to Peggy.

"I wonder what they'll find. I wonder if Mr Adanar will know straight away. Or whether I'll have to wait days for the results?"

Peggy looked at me with her big, wide-open grey eyes, then led me out of the hospital and down the road to the pub where we'd arranged to meet Dave. We pushed our way through the after-work crowd and sat huddled together on three red velvet stools, enveloped in the clouds of smoke and the ceaseless roar of conversation all around us. Dave and Peggy let me do all the talking, allowing me to shed the pent-up emotion of the last two weeks. Now and then they said just the right thing at just the right moment. In just the right way.

I looked at my watch. A whole hour had flown by. "I must go back to the hospital now. I must be there when Andrew comes back from theatre. I must see Mr Adanar."

"We'll be waiting," Dave and Peggy said in unison.

I had more courage now than when I'd left the hospital an hour ago. Dutch, I think they call it.

The nurses at the desk smiled but shook their heads.

"They're not back yet, love."

Why so long, I wondered, as I went into his room to wait.

I gazed down through the double glazed soundproof windows at the aimless noiseless madness of the traffic in the street below. Headlights. Stopping. Starting. Crawling. Darting. Flashing by. Like a scene from an ancient silent movie.

It didn't look real.

And like my own life right now I did not believe that any of this was happening.

At last Mr Adanar came into the room. I turned and blinked at him. I waited for him to speak but all I could hear was a buzzing in my ears and all I could see was an imprint of the maze of headlights from the streets below that were still dancing before my eyes.

Chapter Five

March 1984

Weird atmosphere in theatre. All green.
A jab. A cut. Then nothing.
The night awful.
Kept waking in a daze,
Always thirsty.
Night nurse jabbed me
Three or four times to kill the pain.
Leg all bandaged up. In a mummified way.

Breakfast. Bacon and egg.
Ughh!

At last Mr Adanar's visit.
Found some soft tissue that didn't look promising, he said.
Now I'm really scared cos I guess he'll cut me up again.
Friendly physio brings me crutches.
Walking very painful
But I'm damned if I'm not going to succeed.

- O -

Mr Adanar sits down next to me.

"It is definitely a tumour," he says.

His voice is deep and soothing. His words a panga through my chest.

"But it will be a long time – up to ten days – before any final and positive diagnosis can be made about the exact nature of the tumour."

Is it malignant? I want to scream, but my lips are silent.

"There will be a progressive investigation by the pathologists who

55

will be able to give me the first stage of their results tomorrow. Each day will bring further results until finally, on the tenth day, the results will be conclusive."

Conclusive of what?

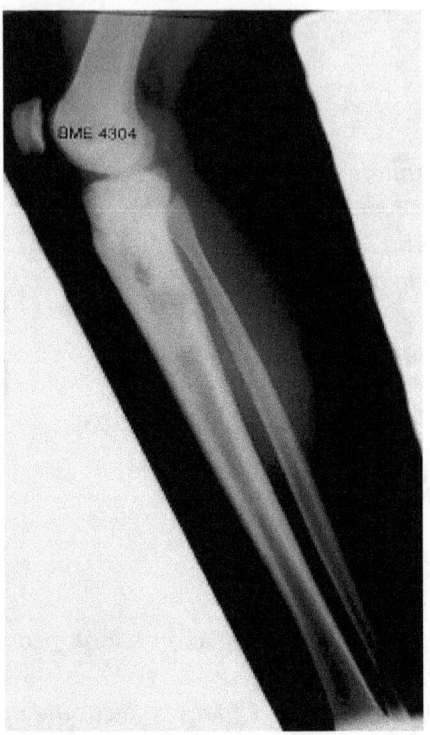

X-Ray of Tumour at top of tibia, 1984.

The question thunders inside my head but on the outside I remain perfectly calm.

He looks at me with his eyes full of compassion though his face retains the mask of his professionalism. "It is likely that I will surgically remove the tumour from the tibia and fill the space with bone which I will take from Andrew's hip. There are many different types of tumour," he explained, "and the treatment will depend on what kind it is and what stage of development it has reached."

His voice comes and goes in waves, as though I am imprisoned in a box beneath the sea.

"But if it is malignant ..." He pauses and I stop breathing.

56

"... I will have to amputate his leg."

I stare at him like a rabbit in the headlights of a car. Paralysed with fear.

Amputate his leg?

Andrew with only one leg?

My young, beautiful, golden haired son.

With only one leg.

And then it dawns on me. He is telling me in the gentlest way he knows how, that my son may have cancer. He doesn't use that word. That dreaded word. They never do. If they said it more freely it would not be so dreaded. They call it all sorts of things.

But never Cancer.

The Big C. It is what happens to other people. Old people. But now it looms large and threateningly into our normal placid lives.

How can an eighteen year old have cancer? What had he done wrong?

A numbness spreads through my body. Oh no! *Not* what had *he* done wrong?

What had *I* done wrong?

I try hard to take in everything Mr Adanar is saying. He is extremely worried and upset. That much I do understand.

"I will phone you tomorrow with the first results," he says. "If at any time you need to speak to me please contact me at my rooms. Or at the hospital. Or at home."

He gives me his home telephone number, something one never normally gets from a busy consultant. Finally he leaves the room and I am left staring at the wall. Face to face with the reality that my son could have a life-threatening illness. I am so frightened for Andrew. I want so badly to take him in my arms and comfort him but he is still in the recovery room and Sister says it would be better if he is left to sleep.

Outside, Dave and Peggy are patiently waiting.

"Are you okay?" Dave asks. He takes my arm.

I shake my head. I cannot speak.

"Come on," he says. "Let's go back to the pub."

- 0 -

Traffic roared. Pavement people jostled and laughed. Lights flashed. It was as though I was not really part of it but in a bubble that separated me from the rest of the world.

Dave and Peggy supported me, one on either side, and gradually the iron band round my throat began to loosen. When at last I could speak I told them in a torrent of incoherent words what Mr Adanar had said.

"And he may have to amputate the leg," I cried at last.

Straight away Peggy phoned Jenny to tell her they were bringing me home. I watched the lights flash by as the taxi sped through Kentish town, Archway and up the hill to Highgate. Outside Jenny's lovely old three-storeyed Victorian house, surrounded by shimmering oaks and overlooking the fairyland of London, I hugged Dave and Peggy. Without their selfless care I could not have coped.

As soon as I got in I phoned Colin. I tried to picture what it must have been like for him, so far away, worrying his head off and not knowing what would happen to his son.

There was a tremor in his voice. "I'll phone every day," he said, and I blew him a kiss down the phone.

Jenny put her arms around me, then opened a bottle of red wine to go with the spaghetti bolognaise she had cooked for supper. Red wine was poison to me, but that night, while into my niece's sympathetic ears I poured out my anguish, I didn't even notice I was drinking it. I had to keep talking and it was so good to talk to Jenny.

The events of the day had taken their toll. Soon I could not keep my eyes open a minute longer. I staggered off to bed and fell into a deep dreamless sleep. Around midnight I awoke, my pulse galloping, my arms numb, my head spinning and my stomach churning.

The house was dark and silent. So as not to wake up the whole household, I avoided the worst of the creaking floor-boards, treading like a chameleon with giant hesitant steps, and somehow I found the bathroom. Fifteen minutes later, weak, shaking and freezing with cold, I stumbled back to bed.

Next morning the au pair girl woke me with a life-saving mug of hot Rooibos tea and at seven-thirty, with my head still pounding from the aftermath of the red wine, I was walking down the steep hill to Highgate Station. Past the quiet happy settled families in their quiet well-tended gardens in their quiet tree-lined speed-bumped street. Past the mini roundabout and the traffic thundering over Archway Road. Down the long slow chunnering escalator to the platform deep below ground level.

The train was already full. I stood all the way to Kings Cross, clinging to the one and only space left on the upright pole and hemmed in like a sardine by an army of silent commuters. I got off at Baker Street into the melee that London's solemn faced workers have to endure every working day of their lives and I thought fleetingly of the wide open spaces of Zambia I had left behind me.

Andrew was still pretty groggy from the anaesthetic and the pain-killing drugs, and I didn't get much sense out of him.

"How do you feel, darling?"

Silly question and I should have known I would receive a silly answer.

"Bloody awful, Mum."

Bone operations are painful, as I knew only too well from my mutilated feet which after all these months were still giving me hell.

I stayed with him all day. I thought how fortunate we were that this bed had been available and that we had private medical insurance – a must when you work in a developing African country where highly specialised medical facilities are often non-existent.

He slept most of the day. I answered the phone calls, received the visitors. But what can you say to people when you know nothing yourself?

And when you dare not even hint at what Mr Adanar has told you it might be.

It was comforting to know that our friends were thinking of him, and so kind of them to phone.

My youngest sister Muriel arrived that day from Zimbabwe to sort out family problems. Aghast at the news about Andrew, she came straight to the hospital to see us. Though we lived in neighbouring African countries we had seen little of each other during the long drawn-out Rhodesian war when the border between Zambia and Zimbabwe was closed.

By nightfall Andrew was still very sleepy. I tucked him in and gave him a kiss, then went home to Jenny's.

After supper I decided to make a phone call.

A phone call which would turn out to be the most important call I would ever make in my life.

To Dr Philip Rodin's wife, Jo.

I had no motive for making the call other than normal social contact with a friend, but I'm sure that subconsciously I needed the support of someone in the medical world although I did not formulate it that way.

We had met the Rodins in Menorca several years ago and liked them. Jo and I had lunched together in Manchester when she gave one of her special nursing lectures on the importance of medical staff involving the parents of sick children in hospital, but otherwise we had not seen much of them outside of Menorca.

Jo answered the phone. As coherently as I could I told her about the bone scan and the bone biopsy and the possible result. Without any histrionics she asked lots of questions and then said she would meet me for lunch on Thursday at Dickins & Jones, the famous Regent Street department store that closed in 2007.

I still had a splitting headache and was about to go to bed when the phone rang.

It was Mr Adanar.

With the promised report on the first lab results.

"Things are not looking good," he said.

- 0 -

Andrew's wound was very painful but he was fed up and bored with being immobile and soon started getting out of bed.

"I shouldn't be here, Mum," he said on the second day. "This place is great. It's friendly. Comfortable. Like a hotel. The nurses and staff are brilliant. It's fantastic, really. A lot of fun." He looked at me and smiled a wistful smile. "But I wish I was at school. Playing in the House First Eleven hockey final."

He managed the crutches very well and by Wednesday was wandering out of his room to talk in his natural gregarious manner to nurses and other patients. I took this opportunity to go shopping for the things Andrew needed. I thought it might take my mind off the waiting but the crowds and the noise and the pain in my feet were suddenly too much. Forcing myself to stop at Marks & Spencer I bought Andrew some shirts and shorts to wear in bed because he hated pyjamas, then hurried back, running through the crowds, frantic in case I had left him alone for too long.

I needn't have worried. The bed was surrounded by visitors and a nurse was putting up another batch of get-well cards.

A few minutes later Mr Adanar phoned with his daily up-date on

60

the results. It was only day three but he sounded disturbed.

I held my breath.

"The pathologists are working on it", he said. "There's still a long way to go but I'm afraid it isn't looking good."

I didn't know what questions to ask so I asked nothing. I said thank you and put down the phone.

- 0 -

The days of that cliff-hanging week were elongated by the necessity to count them. Time spans of interminable length that somehow I had to live through. How, I do not know. Unbelievably it was only Thursday. Day four out of the ten. If you counted Monday.

It was also the day I was having lunch with Jo.

First I went to the hospital. I arrived at eleven. Mr Adanar had already been to see Andrew but I needed to talk to him myself so I rang him from the phone at the end of the fourth floor passage, where I could talk out of Andrew's earshot.

"I'm still waiting for further pathology tests," Mr Adanar said, with the infinite patience that was one of the hallmarks of his care. "So it is not yet possible to make a positive diagnosis." His voice was brimming with compassion – not in the choice of words he used but in the slow, lilting tone of concern and empathy in the way he spoke them.

He must have a son Andrew's age, I suddenly thought. He must know what I'm going through. "We can't hurry this process," he went on, "but I should know more by tomorrow."

Not a glimmer of hope there, but I could not let Andrew see me looking upset so I put a smile on my face and breezed back into his room.

"I'm feeling much better today, Mum," he told me. He was enjoying the hospital social life. He was getting on well with all the Sisters and nurses and had made friends with one or two patients. The free and easy visiting hours allowed a regular flow of friends to his bedside and his phone rang often.

And I had a sneaking feeling he was keen on one of the nurses.

- 0 -

I met Jo for lunch at Dickins & Jones. It was as though I was on a stage

61

set: A busy restaurant scene. Noise. Two people sitting at a table. What would happen next?

After ordering our salad lunch, Jo wasted no time and began to talk to me as no other person had ever done before.

One of Jo's many jobs – missions in life – was to improve, on a national scale, the liaison between the parents of children in hospital, both with their children and with the doctors and nurses who treated them. I was lucky, so very lucky, that there was no other person alive who was better equipped to give me the help she started to give me that day.

First she outlined the things that Andrew might have wrong with him, explaining the different forms of cancer and the many stages of development. How the pathology would soon establish which kind it was – *if* it was malignant – and how those results would determine the treatment.

"It could be osteosarcoma," she said. "A rare, fast growing cancer which normally only strikes teenagers."

I gulped. "I've never heard of it."

"Yes you have. It's what Senator Edward Kennedy's son had."

"Oh, really?"

I swallowed hard. In Zambia we didn't always get world news, but the magazine picture of Kennedy's son with only one leg leapt in front of my eyes, the stump of the other leg hanging useless at its side.

"And Terry Fox too," she added quietly, "who ran across Canada with only one leg to raise funds to fight cancer."

I screwed up my face. What was she trying to tell me? I had seen the film on Zambia Television, but what had the heroic and tragic Terry Fox got to do with my son Andrew? And why had she omitted to remind me that young Terry Fox had died a year later?

"But of course Andrew may not have that," she added hastily, seeing the expression on my face. "It's extremely rare. There are only one or two hundred cases a year in the whole country. Andrew's tumour might even be benign. I'm only telling you the worst possible thing that he could have."

I pursed my lips and breathed in deeply. I tried to convince myself that what Jo was telling me was that it was highly unlikely that Andrew would have this very rare – what was it called? Osteosarcoma?

Or was she?

The waitress removed our half-eaten salads and brought the tea.

The mundane acts reminded me that we were in the real world. Not a stage set. That this was me sitting here at Dickins & Jones. That what Jo Rodin was saying was directed at me. That I was not watching actors in a play.

Jo poured the tea. "It's a very remote possibility," she said. "But if it is osteosarcoma Mr Adanar will have to amputate his leg. You must accept that. It will be to save Andrew's life."

I heard her words. I understood them. But even as she carried on speaking I could not believe they applied to me.

"You will have to be very strong in order to support Andrew throughout the treatment. He will be angry at first. Frustrated. He will often vent his anger on you and will sometimes reject you, but only because there will be no-one else he can do it to. You are only at the beginning of a period in your life which will make more demands on you as a mother than at any other time."

I opened my mouth. She touched my hand to silence me.

"But don't worry. You will cope. In fact you will cope without ever wavering. With great strength and fortitude. I know you will."

My mouth twisted into a disbelieving smile. I had hardly touched my tea and as I pushed my cup to one side Jo completed her counselling.

"And after it's all over you will probably have a nervous breakdown!"

She laughed. And I laughed too. Because I was the last person in the whole wide world who could ever have a nervous breakdown.

- 0 -

Early next morning before work, Jo visited Andrew to have a chat with him on his own. When I saw him later I could see that intermingled with her indomitable light banter which was always guaranteed to cheer him up she must also have contrived to secrete into his unsuspecting mind the seeds of her special brand of support.

"I'm in the best possible hands, you know, Mum. I've got nothing to be scared of. As long as I just keep being strong."

- 0 -

While Andrew remained unaware of the unfolding drama in his midst,

63

the nursing staff were acutely conscious of the tightrope he was walking. They were always popping in and out so there was seldom a moment during the day when he had time to reflect on the outcome of the tests he knew were being carried out in order to determine the kind of treatment he would receive. Late at night, though, he was alone, with plenty of time to think.

This was when nurse Laura, then on night duty, came in on the scene.

She was the one on the spot when the final diagnosis was revealed to him so unexpectedly and so starkly in the middle of the night. She held his hand. She comforted him. She fell in love with him and inevitably Andrew fell for her too.

Chapter Six

I try hard not to count the days but they tick themselves off in large red letters in my mind. Mr Adanar said he would have news today, but whenever I phone his rooms he is somewhere else.

At last, at five-thirty, using the phone at the end of the passage on the fourth floor, I catch him at his surgery.

"It is now almost certain that it is osteosarcoma. This means I will have to amputate the leg."

I hear Mr Adanar's voice but not his words.

My limbs are numb.

My body floats away.

I am drowning in a sea of terror.

I look around for a life-line and miraculously at that moment Jo pops her head around the corner. I beckon her. Gaze into her diamond bright eyes. Speechless.

She grabs the phone. Says hello to Mr Adanar. Shoos me away.

I totter backwards and forwards like a headless chicken, up and down the corridor outside Andrew's room. Terrified of going in because I don't know what to say or how to say it and he will know anyway, by taking one look at me, ashen faced and wild eyed, that something is catastrophically wrong.

- O -

Jo finally put down the phone. She led me to an empty room and pushed me into a chair. She sat down opposite me and took both my hands in hers.

"Mr Adanar is now ninety-nine percent certain of the diagnosis," she said, her voice steady, calm and quiet. "But he can only make his final decision on Wednesday. On day ten. When the diagnosis will be a hundred percent positive. He will amputate Andrew's leg next Friday."

The walls tilted towards me. I stared at Jo. She squeezed my hands.

"It's drastic, I know. But if he's going to save Andrew's life he must operate immediately. Every day the tumour is growing larger. The possibility of it spreading is increasing. He's considered other methods of treatment but is convinced that amputation is the only way of making sure that Andrew lives."

My head reeled.

What would this do to Andrew?

How would such an active, sport-loving young man cope with only one leg? I covered my face with my hands. Oh my God! How will he fly a plane with only one leg? How will he become a pilot? The only thing he so passionately wants to do with his life?

I pictured him sitting alone with his cello, day after day, month after month, year after year, looking longingly out of the window, the slow, sad notes filling the silent air.

"And who is going to tell him?" I asked, fearing it would have to be me as I was his mother.

"Mr Adanar will tell him tomorrow morning," she answered gently. She is a mother too, I thought. She must know how difficult this would be. She understands. "And immediately afterwards he will talk to both of you together so that Andrew will know that you are also fully in the picture. That way, there will never be any necessity to hide anything from each other."

I nodded, wondering if this gem of an idea was Jo's, almost certain that it was.

Suddenly I remembered my husband. "What about Colin? He'll also have to be told."

Already I could feel the now familiar band tightening around my throat and doubted I'd be capable of this when he rang me tonight. In any case, I still couldn't assimilate all the detail. Only one terrible thing was clear.

Jo read my mind. "When Colin phones you tonight, ask him to ring me. I'll tell him. As kindly as I can." She took a deep breath. She had a special rapport with Colin. I was confident she would do it better than anyone else I knew.

She helped me to my feet. "You're not eating properly. Just look at you," she said. "Skin and bone."

She faced me squarely, forced me to look at her. "You're going to need all the strength you have. You'll have to call on all your reserves. If you don't look after yourself you could become ill." She shook her head. "A proper diet and enough sleep are a must."

At the nurses' desk she asked the Sister to give me a few sleeping tablets, angry that throughout this fraught period my well-being had been totally ignored by all the medical staff. She promised to ask Philip to prescribe some more for me.

But we had Andrew to think about now, so we breezed in to have a little chat with him, pretending that nothing was wrong.

Jo did most of the talking. I sat there with my whole being screeching to throw my arms around my son and tell him everything will be all right, darling, because no matter what happens we'll take care of you and love you ... But I must stay calm. I must let things happen Mr Adanar's way and Jo's way. I must smile and I must move slowly and calmly as I always do instead of giving way to my first instincts to throw myself on the ground and scream and beat my chest with my fists ...

Jo and I left the hospital at half-past six, going our separate ways. I got to Jenny's just in time for Peter's unexpected arrival from Manchester with his attractive brown-eyed fiancée, Andrea.

And just in time for Colin's call from Zambia.

We talked as strangers. "Things are not good," I told Colin haltingly, "but why don't you phone Jo. She knows more about these medical matters than I do."

Coward!

As I put down the phone I knew that my very lack of words had fuelled his smouldering doubts. If ever we needed to be together it was now. By himself in Lusaka, he was probably in a worse state of tension than I was. Even though the possibility of malignancy had been uppermost in my mind I had still not uttered this fear to him, but I was sure that by now he must have guessed.

My heart was breaking for him. How would he take the news which at this very moment he was hearing from Jo? He is a decisive man. A man of action. Not afraid of the truth.

I shuddered to think what he would do.

After a quick supper we took a taxi back to the hospital and Andrew was delighted to see his brother and his future sister-in-law. I found it hard to speak normally so I let Peter and his equally articulate Andrea do most of the talking. Lawyers are clever with words.

My three sons were alike in looks, with their penetrating blue eyes and their blond hair and their warm, ready smiles, but every time I looked at Andrew I got a sick, numb feeling. He looked so well that I

67

found it impossible to equate his youth and vitality with the threat which now hung over his life.

At ten o'clock we kissed him good night and trooped silently out. Back in Highgate I took one of the sleeping pills and went straight to bed, but just as I was dropping off the phone rang.

It was Colin in Zambia. The line was faint and crackling as usual, but just clear enough to make out that Jo had told him everything.

He was in a state of shock.

"Have you told Andrew?" he asked, his tone threateningly sharp.

I swallowed hard. "No."

The line crackled with another burst of machine gun fire.

"Why not?" he demanded. His voice was harsh yet strangely muffled.

"It's not for us to break the news before the surgeon does," I shouted, guiltily telling myself that I was his mother and should indeed be the one to do this.

The line crackled again. I heard Colin grunt incoherently and then there was a click. I put down the phone. My eyes closed, the lids heavy from the sleeping pill, and in a few minutes I was asleep.

But not for long.

- 0 -

I hear the ringing in my sleep. I snap on the light. Five-thirty! Who on earth can it be so early? I grab the phone.

"Mum! They're going to cut off my leg!"

My blood runs cold. "Oh my darling . . ."

"Dad phoned. He said they're going to cut off my leg!"

"It'll be all right, Andrew. We'll be there as soon as we can."

It will be all right.

Useless, vacant words and I am sickened that I cannot say or do anything more. "I love you, darling," is all I manage to say.

I put down the phone, feeling my armour begin to crack as momentarily I give way to an involuntary torrent of tears. Tears of frustration. Of desperately wanting to help him. Of wanting to make it all go away but knowing that I can't.

Pull yourself together, woman! Jo said you had to be strong.

Peter emerges from his bedroom. Bleary eyed. Bewildered.

"What's going on?" he asks.

68

Dry eyed now, I tell him.

"Oh my God!" he murmurs, then hugs me so tightly that I almost give way again.

The au pair girl makes tea and toast while I phone Mr Adanar to tell him what has happened, then Jenny drives us all to the hospital.

Andrew is frightened, angry and morose, but at first seems more concerned about his father than himself.

"Poor Dad," he says when we are all gathered round him. "What a thing to hear when he was all on his own. You should have heard him, Mum. He was so upset. I've never heard him like that before. It's not fair."

Stunned into silence I let Peter do most of the talking. Right now I am too involved, too much a part of Andrew. Peter can be detached. With his lawyer's skills he can choose the right words.

"Andrew," he says calmly. "It won't be the end of the world to have only one leg, you know. Look at Grandpa. And Douglas Bader. They had none." He is only too aware of Andrew's passionate dream to become a pilot.

Andrew stares out of the window. He looks up at the sky.

"Yes. I know, Pete. But when Bader flew with no legs they were short of pilots. It was a long time ago. In the war. Things are different now. The RAF will never take me now. Not with only one leg. I won't be able to take up that wonderful scholarship now ..."

My heart contracts with sadness and with pity. It is too terrible to imagine him being robbed of his chance to fulfil his dream before he has even started.

Then he says something which takes my breath away.

"It's a funny thing, you know, Pete. But I'd already had a strange feeling that I might lose my leg."

- 0 -

Although at first Andrew was hurt, shocked, horrified, frightened and bewildered, in the end I think that hearing the news the way he did made him acutely aware of the very worst he thought could happen, and straight away he began to prepare for it.

Jo's counselling came into its own now. She had warned me that he would be angry. Angry at the whole world because there was no one single person he could blame for what had happened to him.

69

"But you can't vent your anger on the whole world," she had said. "You have to vent it on someone. He can't risk showing his anger to his brothers or to his friends. Instinctively he knows this would endanger their love for him. But subconsciously he knows that no matter what he does or says to you, nothing will make you love him any less. Because you're his mother. So that someone will have to be you."

And so it was.

As the weeks went by he became bad-tempered and irritable and rude. It came as a shock at first, but because of Jo's priceless advice I could understand it. Each little knock jolted me, but left me intact.

"He's also very frightened," I told Jo during one of our tête-à-tête sessions. "Though he's never said as much to me, I can sense it."

Jo thought about this for a moment, then nodded. "He's frightened of losing his physical wholeness," she said, feeling for her words as though this was a brand new theory she had just conceived. "Frightened of becoming less than a man. At eighteen years old the physical is all important. It's part of the reason for being, with the sexual drive at its peak and physical attractiveness part of the process of sexual achievement. To lose a part of his body which would leave him unattractive to the opposite sex would at this stage mean an end to his very reason for being alive."

- 0 -

It is a strangely quiet Saturday afternoon in the hospital. The visitors have all gone home, many of the other patients Andrew knows have left, and there is even a lull in the usual steady stream of phone calls. Andrew looks at me sullenly.

"Let's go for a walk, Mum."

I shake my head.

"Please, Mum ..." His voice has a beseeching lilt, difficult to deny.

It is an unusually warm spring day and the nurses say he can go. So, wearing only the little shorts and shirt he is wearing in bed, and armed with his crutches, he and I venture into the hustle and bustle of the London streets.

Suddenly Andrew stops. A young man is running towards us on the opposite side of the road. Leaning on his crutches Andrew watches him.

"That should be me! That will never be me! I'll never be able to do

70

that again! I'm a cripple!" he shouts, and there is thunder in his eyes.

At last it has sunk in. At last the floodgates have been opened. And in the impersonal privacy of the busy street the anger begins to gush forth from his wounded spirit.

"I'll never play hockey again. Or squash. Or golf. I'll never run again. Or fly a plane. Oh, Mum! Why?"

Although he is talking to me I realise he is really talking to the world. He is looking all around him. He is shouting at the top of his voice but he doesn't care and I don't care either and I want to shout with him.

"Why? Why? Why me?" he implores.

I feel the pain of the injustice too, but I am glad he is no longer bottling up his feelings.

We turn the corner and see the Parish Church. The long wide steps leading to the entrance are too steep for Andrew on crutches but he stops at the foot of them and gazes upwards.

He stands perfectly still.

"Where are you, God?" he says quietly.

I stand equally still, oblivious to the chatter of the passing people, the roar of traffic, the flutter of pigeons' wings. What, I wonder, is going through his mind? Fear? Despair? Hope?

Or merely anger, knowing he will never run again?

He turns to me then looks up at the church. "When I can walk better I'm going to come back here and take communion." Seldom have I seen such passion and fire in his eyes.

We had not brought Andrew up to be religious. My father had been the eldest son in a long line of ministers of the church, but had rebelled during his Theology degree course at Aberdeen University and changed to Philosophy and Psychology, never to be forgiven by his father. My mother was also raised as a devout Christian, and had also undergone her own quiet transition. So, although neither of my parents subscribed to any actual religion, I had the benefit of all the 'good' things Christians are taught, which in turn I passed on to my sons.

Yet right now Andrew looks to me like someone to whom God is reaching out.

But what is He thinking of? I ask myself. Why is He making Andrew suffer? Why has He done this to Andrew?

I look at my son standing motionless at the bottom of the steps,

71

leaning on his crutches, looking upwards.

What has Andrew done to deserve this?

No. I shake my head. Not God. Not Andrew.

Me!

What have I done?

I scroll my memory for any transgression during my pregnancy or in Andrew's early years, attributable to me, but can think of none.

I look upwards too, and in the moment of stillness, with the early spring sunshine irradiating the rich brown bricks of the church, I pray for my son to be saved.

Chapter Seven

The terrible shock to Andrew of the impending amputation quite overshadowed for him the fact that he had cancer. Right now losing a limb was far more threatening.

As Jo had said, it was the threat to his masculinity that was the biggest danger.

Only later did I learn that after Colin's devastating phone call on Friday night Laura had comforted him. With her gentle voice and soft brown eyes and tresses of gossamer auburn hair, she had overstepped her normal duties as a nurse and had told him when he had most needed to hear it that even though he would soon have only one leg, he was still physically attractive.

He had badly needed to know this, though when she confessed to me that she had given him a hug that night I was initially a little bit shocked, yet later I realised the value of what had happened.

Over the months to come she played another important role. She filled a social gap created by the isolation of his illness, which left Andrew on one side as the condemned patient, and his many visitors on the other; some who were unaccountably embarrassed and could no longer act naturally in his presence. Laura cut right through that barrier and treated him as if he were quite normal.

She was an excellent nurse. Efficient, diligent, caring and compassionate. She had a terrific sense of humour. I was fond of her and we got on very well, though with a certain wariness on each side that was difficult to define. Sometimes I caught her looking at me in an odd manner, almost as though she felt I was in the way.

Now and then I would watch them together. I thought that perhaps she was a few years older than him, not many, not enough to detract from her freshness and youth but enough to give her sufficient maturity to be slotted into a rack slightly above that of mere girl-friend.

"She's fantastic, Mum" Andrew said to me one day. "So strong willed. And you know what? She wants to join the Royal Air Force!"

Ah! So was that part of the attraction, I wondered. A kindred spirit?

One afternoon I deliberately left the hospital in order to give Andrew a break from my constant presence and give him and Laura a chance to talk.

I walked aimlessly down Oxford Street, my still wonky feet shooting arrows of pain up my legs. With empty eyes I gazed into the myriad shop windows and listened with deaf ears to the hum of humanity jostling its way down the busy street with its never-ending stream of bright red buses and nimble black taxis.

Why am I doing this? I asked myself. *Andrew is my son. I want to be with him all the time, care for him, love him. Why should I delegate this to some other woman, even for just a few hours?*

Was I becoming jealous?

Heaven forbid. I had heard of mothers who were, but it was unthinkable that I could be like them.

- 0 -

To break the tedium of the hospital bed, Mr Adanar agreed to a day out on Sunday. Peter had been granted indefinite compassionate leave by the firm of solicitors he worked for in Manchester, and after we'd seen his fiancée Andrea off at Euston Station we drove Andrew to Farnborough to see Emily, the girl he'd had lunch with the day before he was admitted to hospital. She was a special friend of his, one of a group of girls from a neighbouring girls-only school who always came to the Bradfield College dances. She was only seventeen but full of empathy and concern, and while the rest of us talked in hushed tones she spent the entire two hours staring into Andrew's eyes and whispering sweet nothings in his ear. Emily's parents seemed somewhat ill at ease, and lunch was a subdued affair. They were clearly not happy about their only daughter's obvious infatuation with someone whose future was so uncertain.

Later we drove to Bradfield College and Andrew savoured the unscheduled gift of a few hours to spend with his best friends, Simon, Stuart and James. Underneath his spirited façade he was very emotional, and so were the boys; they seemed stunned by the news as though they could not believe this was happening to their mate.

- 0 -

The following morning at half-past six Peter and I were standing at the barrier at Heathrow's Terminal Three, anxiously scanning the stream of bleary-eyed passengers wheeling their luggage through the Customs exit door.

An hour later Colin appeared, looking distressed and tired after a sleepless ten hour flight from Lusaka. We drove straight to the hospital and I watched him fight back his tears as he and Andrew sat on the bed, locked in each other's arms.

They talked for many hours, and with his father's stoic inspiration it was soon obvious that Andrew had begun to face up to his ordeal.

Colin is a very positive pragmatic person with both feet firmly on the ground. I had been existing in a vacuum of unreality and fear but with my husband's arrival I became aware of the many practical things that had to be done.

"We can't go on staying with Jenny," he announced at lunch time, "in spite of her extremely kind offer. Besides, we must be nearer the hospital."

That very afternoon he went flat hunting and quickly decided on a huge sixth floor apartment next to the Planetarium in the Baker Street Underground Station complex. It had once been very grand but now its furnishings were a bit tatty and worn. It was convenient, and if necessary could accommodate all the family and some friends too. We decided to move in the following morning.

In the meantime the most significant event in Andrew's life occurred.

Late that afternoon on our way out of the hospital we found Philip Rodin waiting to see us.

Philip had been quietly keeping an eye on the events of the past week. He had stayed well in the background, but when he heard about Mr Adanar's planned amputation in a few days' time, he moved to centre stage.

He had spent from Friday night until Monday afternoon making enquiries amongst colleagues and medical acquaintances throughout London.

"I wanted the aggressive decision to amputate a teenager's leg to be backed by a second opinion," he told us. "Not any second opinion. But the best one there is."

Philip read a lot. He was obsessed with keeping up with the giant leaps being made daily in the field of medicine and always had his medical ear to the ground. Recently he had read about a new treatment for osteosarcoma. This was far removed from his own field of expertise, but as an eminent physician at a London hospital he was in an excellent position to learn from his colleagues that amputation – the previous one-and-only treatment for osteosarcoma – had indeed recently been augmented by a revolutionary new treatment, still in the experimental stages.

"Instead of amputation," Philip said in his calm, gentle voice, "the affected bones can be replaced with a metal prosthesis made of titanium." His lean face was alive with enthusiasm, his dark almond shaped eyes dancing with excitement. "And this would be combined with powerful new chemotherapy treatment –"

He paused, then leaned forward, his pale cheeks suddenly taking on an unaccustomed glow. His voice wavered with emotion. "— not just *after* surgery ..." He looked triumphantly from Colin to me. "... but before surgery as well!"

Philip had also ascertained that undoubtedly the best authority on this was a pioneer of the operation, Mr Rodney Sweetnam, (later Sir Rodney and from 1995 – 1998 President of the Royal College of Surgeons and former Orthopaedic Surgeon to the Queen) who led a team based at The Middlesex Hospital in London.

We sat on the edge of our chairs, open-mouthed and speechless with excitement.

"It won't be a straightforward business to obtain Mr Sweetnam's opinion, let alone get him to take the case," Philip explained, shaking his head, and in spite of his exultation allowing his patrician features to reflect his anxiety. "Time is short so you must talk to Mr Adanar as soon as possible, Colin, and tell him you would like a second opinion."

"How can we do that?" Colin asked, unaccustomed to the intricacies of medical etiquette. "I've never been in a position before where it was necessary to seek a second opinion."

"It's something people should do more often," Philip said. "That and making sure they get the best surgeon for the job. Tell him you've heard about this new treatment and that you understand Mr Sweetnam is the man doing this work. Ask him if he would mind calling Mr Sweetnam in for a second opinion. And then hope that he'll take over the case," he added grimly. "Medical etiquette unfortunately prevents us from making a direct approach to Mr Sweetnam."

76

Colin and I felt light-headed with hope and expectation. We could hardly believe what we were hearing. If it really was possible, it would be a miracle.

Colin went immediately to see Mr Adanar. Following Philip's instruction to the letter he explained that he had heard about the alternative treatment. Mr Adanar was in the middle of a long list of patients but promised to contact Colin as soon as possible.

It was sheer chance that we knew the Rodins. We had met on an almost deserted beach on Colom – a tiny uninhabited island off the north-east coast of Menorca. By a happy coincidence we had bumped into them again at a country restaurant, where we had sat under the stars eating barbecued prawns and drinking wine and watching the moonlight play on the dazzling white walls of the ancient farmhouse.

It was sheer chance too that after Andrew's first consultation with Mr Adanar, I had phoned Jo for a chat.

Not chance though, that Philip was so conscientious.

It was difficult not to question why Philip, who was not even remotely connected with orthopaedic surgery, should be aware of new ground being broken in the field of osteosarcoma, with limbs and lives being saved, while others were so set on amputation.

Andrew needed to have his mind taken off the impending amputation and I was thankful that a host of visitors arrived that evening.

"Let's all go to Muswells," Colin suggested, and proceeded to lead the motley crowd down the narrow streets to the nearby trendy restaurant. There was a convivial mood amongst the large gathering of family, friends and nurses, all striving to keep Andrew's spirits high. It was artificial I know, but the last thing he needed was to see long, miserable faces all around him.

We had our own spirits to keep up too. Somehow we had to try to relieve the unbearable tension of not knowing whether Mr Adanar would agree to open Philip's new magical door and if he did, whether Mr Sweetnam would take on the case.

- 0 -

Next morning we moved to our rented flat next to the Planetarium, regretfully leaving Jenny whose distinct brand of caring and unstinting help was so special.

Peter was still with us, and though filled with hope and anticipation the three of us were in an explosive state of suspense as we waited to hear from Mr Adanar.

"Come on," Peter said as soon as we had unpacked. "We can't hang around here all day. Let's go to the hospital. Mr Adanar might not even phone today."

As we walked into Andrew's room the phone rang. It was Mr Adanar for Colin.

Peter and I held our breath. We had not spoken to Andrew about Philip's intervention in case it came to nothing. We watched Colin's face closely. He nodded a few times, said thank you very much and put down the phone.

Then he grinned. Peter and I were frantic with curiosity.

"*What?*" we said in unison.

Colin looked at us, savouring the moment. "Mr Sweetnam is coming to see you tomorrow, Andrew. To look at your leg."

Andrew looked puzzled. "Who's Mr Sweetnam?"

Colin explained who he was but not any details of why he was being consulted. It would not do to raise his hopes.

That evening we found ourselves again at Muswells, with family and faithful friends, Laura of course, and two other nurses as well. After the meal the nurses asked if Andrew could go with them to a night club.

Colin, Peter and I looked at each other dubiously.

Laura whispered in my ear. "A sort of last fling with both his legs intact."

I was horrified at the very thought.

"Please," Laura said.

"Okay," Colin said, and off they all went.

He wasn't very popular with the night staff when he arrived back in his hospital room at two o'clock the following morning, but it all helped to take his mind off his forthcoming ordeal.

That night in bed the agony of not knowing ate like acid into the fabric of my mind, shredding it into a maelstrom of tattered thoughts.

What would be the outcome of Philip's unexpected intervention?

And had the wheels of medical science turned quickly enough to save Andrew's life?

- 0 -

I awoke at dawn on Wednesday morning with a floating feeling as though I was drifting inside a large bubble in space. I was caught up in a web of fate over which I had no control, but surely there was something I could do. I couldn't just lie back like this and not do anything to save my son.

I telephoned Mr Adanar in the faint hope that there might be some news. Patiently he told me his decision would only be made after Mr Sweetnam's visit and after the pathologist's results were in his hands. On Thursday. The tenth day. The day the pathologist's final verdict was due.

Then he said something which made my blood run cold.

"However, I already know what I want to do, and as far as I'm concerned I have not changed my mind."

I shivered as I put down the phone. I knew exactly what he meant.

An hour later the phone rang. It was Andrew. He was half screaming, half crying and I feared the worst. He kept saying the same incoherent thing over and over again, and finally the words began to make sense.

"They're *not* going to cut off my leg! They're *not* going to cut off my leg!"

Then I realised it was laughter I was hearing, not crying. Or maybe it was a mixture of both.

I closed my eyes and gripped the phone tightly.

"That's wonderful, Andrew. We'll be over in a few minutes."

I put down the phone. I was shaking all over.

"*Col! Peter! Come quickly!*" I yelled.

But before leaving for the hospital we quickly phoned Colin Junior in Zambia, who all those miles away was frantic with worry, and then Philip and Jo, and they all screamed with delight.

When we arrived at the hospital there was almost an air of festivity on the fourth floor, so great was everyone's relief. Andrew was sitting up in bed grinning from ear to ear, rejoicing in his reprieve.

"He was great, Dad. He just breezed in, smiling and chatting all the time. Examined me and told me straight away I could have a new metal knee and a new metal tibia and a bit of my femur to replace the bits damaged by the tumour. But the leg will still be mine! My own flesh and blood! A leg that I won't have to take off every night."

When the final pathology results at last confirmed the diagnosis of

79

osteosarcoma, the blow was softened by Mr Adanar's confirmation that he would now carry out the new treatment pioneered by Mr Sweetnam, instead of amputating the leg. Andrew was so elated that even the thought of the big operation did not upset him.

Not then, anyway.

But now a new regime began, and Mr Adanar's orders were clear:

No gallivanting.

Stay in bed.

Lots of rest, and no weight-bearing whatsoever on the leg.

With the immediate emergency over Peter went back to Manchester, to Andrea and to his clients. He is a very affectionate son. He is also very level-headed and calm. With our dynamic eldest son Colin five thousand miles away in Zambia we relied a lot on Peter for the moral support so essential in a family crisis.

"I'll miss you," I said, clinging to him as he boarded the train at Euston Station.

- 0 -

Things were moving fast and when Colin asked Mr Adanar what everything would cost we were staggered at the figure of fifty-five thousand pounds. In 1984 this was a lot of money. Colin spent hours with his calculator and on the phone trying to sort out how we would pay for it all.

The two medical insurance companies which covered Andrew, one through the school, the other through the mining company, supplied Colin with figures showing how much they usually paid out for various treatments and operations. Osteosarcoma was not even listed. It was far too rare. Even straight-forward knee replacements were virtually unknown, and this new treatment was still experimental. They said they couldn't pay anything near that sum, even if they combined their benefits.

So what on earth were we to do?

- 0 -

Early on Friday morning the phone rang. Colin answered. It was the hospital. My heart stopped beating.

"Don't panic," Colin said. "They're only asking us to come over for a meeting with Dr Jelliffe."

Dr Jelliffe, we discovered later, was a highly regarded oncologist brought in by Mr Adanar on the recommendation of Mr Sweetnam to manage the chemotherapy Andrew would receive in conjunction with the surgery to save his leg.

We liked him immediately. Putting us at ease in a comfortable consulting room on the ground floor, he told us he'd already had a chat with Andrew.

"He's taking it wonderfully well," he said, then proceeded to put us in the picture.

"Osteosarcoma is a very rare form of bone cancer," he explained. "Only two out of every one million people world-wide develop the disease but those who do are nearly all between the ages of seven and eighteen.

"A few years ago Andrew's chances of survival would have been a mere fifteen percent," he told us gravely, "with no choice other than amputation. Now, with this new treatment, his chances are eighty-five percent." We learned later that this was only the case if the disease was caught early enough.

I glanced at Colin. It was clear from the expression on his face that he too had no idea that the chances of Andrew surviving had been so low. I thought chillingly that if Philip had not intervened that might still have been the case, and shuddered inwardly when I remembered that today was Friday – the day the amputation was to have been carried out.

We listened in awe as Dr Jelliffe described how they would plan a course of chemotherapy to attack the tumour, specially designed for Andrew.

"The cytotoxic drugs kill rapidly dividing cells, but as they do not kill cancer cells alone and are toxic to normal tissues, we have to be very careful in their use.

"First there will be several treatments of chemotherapy for a period of two and a half months. These are planned to shrink the tumour and at the same time kill any cancer cells which may already have spread to other parts of the body, in particular to the lungs."

Ah! Now I knew why they X-rayed Andrew's lungs the day he had the bone scan. They'd had their suspicions then, so what was all that terrifying poppycock about Paget's disease all about? Or had that first orthopaedic man been as much out of touch as the impression he gave me at the time?

"The lungs are most vulnerable in this rare bone cancer because the fast growing cancer cells are spread by being showered into the bloodstream," he explained. "These cells are then filtered by the small blood vessels in the lungs and any microscopic seeds of cells which might become trapped in the lungs as the blood passes through them could metastasise – grow into secondary tumours. So, by giving chemotherapy treatment *before* the surgery we will be increasing Andrew's chances of survival by more than fifty percent, because the chemotherapy drugs will not only shrink the tumour but hopefully they'll kill any cancer cells which might already have escaped into the bloodstream."

This all sounded too good to be true, but at the same time it was a shock to have it all spelled out to us. Before this we had known only that Andrew might have 'cancer', without any knowledge of what this meant.

"Mr Adanar will then perform the surgery to remove the tumour, replacing the knee and the tibia and part of the femur with a metal prosthesis made from cobalt and titanium. He will probably do the operation in June. Then there'll be a further two and a half months of chemotherapy. Altogether it will take about six months."

Colin and I sought each other's eyes for reassurance and smiled with relief.

An eighty-five percent chance of survival!

Instead of fifteen percent.

Yet to me, these figures were pretty meaningless. Was Dr Jelliffe telling us that even with this magical new treatment our son might still die? Eighty-five percent was not one hundred percent. What about the remaining fifteen percent?

Would Andrew be one of those?

I had a numb feeling about the whole thing, as if he were talking about someone else's son. Not our Andrew.

Dr Jelliffe was mild mannered and charming, with smiling eyes and a slow, measured way of moving and speaking. A man of middle age whose patients' mental well-being was clearly one of his top priorities. Thoughtful in everything he said and did, he had already begun to organise some of the practical things which had to be done before the treatment began.

"Chemotherapy unfortunately has several rather unpleasant side

82

effects," he told us. "I'm afraid one of these is that he is likely to lose his hair. He might also feel very sick."

Dr Jelliffe had such a kind, gentle voice that what he was telling us didn't seem so bad. Nothing compared to losing a leg.

"Two other side effects could be an impairment of hearing. And sterility."

I expect it was the expression of horror on my face that made him momentarily pause.

"So," he said, even more gently, "I've arranged for tests to be carried out this afternoon at The Middlesex Hospital, since these facilities are not available here in this small private hospital."

I felt complete confidence in Dr Jelliffe and that evening I looked up the word 'oncologist.' I couldn't find the word oncology in the small pocket dictionary I always carried with me, but I looked for it in a medical book and found that it means 'the study of tumours', derived from the Greek word oncos, meaning a lump. The oncologist specialises in the treatment of cancer with drugs.

The Middlesex Hospital was a grand old 1930's building in Mortimer Street, in the heart of the West End of London, first opened in 1757, rebuilt in 1935, closed in 2005 and sadly demolished in 2008. Set back from the road, with a car park in its three-sided front courtyard, the imposing pillared portico reflected the building's bygone architectural glory. Despite lack of NHS funds for structural improvements it had retained its extremely high standards of medicine and was a world leader in medical research.

After Andrew's audiogram was completed we were sent to see the man in charge of the sperm bank in the department where they worked on embryos. Handing us a sterile bottle, he asked for a sample to be brought to the lab as soon as possible. If it were found to be worth storing they would then require four more samples before the chemotherapy started in a week's time.

As we went down in the lift Andrew looked at me and grinned. "Well, how about that? At least I'll still be able to be a dad!"

Back in the private hospital, Andrew had a series of blood tests the following morning in preparation for the forthcoming treatment. At three o'clock he was temporarily discharged and told to be back on the third of April, when the chemotherapy was due to start.

We hardly saw him that weekend. When he wasn't with Laura he was talking to friends from all over England, Scotland and Zambia who phoned to wish him good luck.

- 0 -

The nagging problem of how we were going to pay for everything continued to fill Colin's hours with endless calculations. Philip and Jo had been urging us to accept the National Health Service for Andrew's treatment because of the far larger range of medical facilities available in the major London hospitals, and on their next visit to the flat they continued their efforts.

"You only pay for frills in the private hospitals," said down-to-earth Jo, her lively face devoid of its usual merriment.

"You must understand that it is imperative to have the best possible treatment," Philip stressed.

"And major surgery shouldn't be performed at all in small private hospitals, no matter how good they are," said Jo, outspoken as usual.

"Because the NHS is free, many people undervalue its services," said Philip, whose vital work at one of the big hospitals in London had given him a world-wide reputation.

We listened to their advice, were grateful for it as always, yet clung doggedly to the assumption that if you are paying a lot of money for something it must be the best.

On Sunday Laura invited Andrew for lunch at her little bed-sit in Kensington. Colin and I were apprehensive about the leg, afraid that if he fell he might fracture it. He was still unsteady after the biopsy, and the tibia was extremely fragile now, but we needn't have worried; Laura looked after him well and delivered him back to the flat in one piece.

- 0 -

On Monday I took the first sperm sample to The Middlesex Hospital.

The technician took it away while I waited on a wooden bench in the passage, slightly bewildered by my unusual errand. Andrew's life was threatened and here I was on a mission to preserve part of him for posterity. Part of him that was capable of becoming another person before I even knew whether he himself would survive.

Dr Jelliffe's optimism struck me as most significant. He was looking to the future.

84

I bit my lip as I sat staring at the blank wall in front of me.

Would there be a future? I wondered.

The lab technician came back smiling.

"It's a very good sample," he said, then handed me a fresh bottle and asked for four more samples before the chemo began.

"But I must point out," he said firmly, "that if ever these are needed – that is, if your son remains sterile after the chemotherapy – then the artificial insemination will have to take place here at The Middlesex Hospital, where the sperm is stored."

"I don't think that'll be a problem," I murmured, smiling and trying hard to take all this in. Andrew was eighteen. Still at school. Barely a man. Yet the technician was talking about an unknown woman in the future who might bear our grandchild from the sperm I had just carried in a bottle half way across London.

Chapter Eight

March – April 1984

For the next week Colin took over the management of Andrew's days.

The calendar was full of appointments. A nuclear scan; X-rays of the chest, kidneys and liver; another blood test; and measurements and special X-rays of the tibia, knee and femur at the London Orthopaedic Hospital, necessary for the accurate construction of the complicated metal prosthesis which would replace the bones they would remove in June.

The first appointment was at the Hammersmith Hospital for the nuclear scan – the NMR, which stands for Nuclear Magnetic Resonance.

From Andrew's diary:

> It was not too pleasant, almost like falling asleep on an aircraft with the air conditioning blowing in your face. It lasted two hours, which meant that I couldn't phone Laura. I tried but it was too late. I feel awful now. Ever since I've known her, I've either seen her or spoken to her every day. God, how I miss her.

Colin was astonished by this fantastic machine, costing over a million pounds, which picks out clearly, by magnetic resonance, abnormal and diseased cancer tissue.

While they were out, Andrew's friend Simon phoned, anxious about Andrew. Then his cousin Timothy brought a pile of books from the library, all about cancer. Jo popped in later and sifted through the pile, leaving only two for Andrew to read.

"The others are not appropriate at this stage," she said. "They might upset him unnecessarily."

Jo's guidance, as usual, was invaluable.

Philip also called in after he had finished at his rooms in Harley

86

Street and they stayed for hours talking to us. Once again they tried to make us see that Andrew should have his treatment under the NHS.

"You see," Philip said, in his quiet, reserved voice, "because Andrew has a very complicated illness, his treatment will be very specialised."

He was a small slender man with tell-tale eyes that revealed his innate compassion, and a liquid smile that transformed his smooth sensitive face into a sea of undulating creases, each one exposing the underlying deep concern he had, not only for his patients but for his friends who all instinctively knew he would help them.

"There are so many things that could go wrong with the operation," he said. "In a large NHS hospital there'd be an experienced team of experts on hand, ready to deal with any emergency."

- 0 -

Sometimes one's clearest thoughts come out of nowhere in the middle of the night. Long before the roar of Tuesday morning's traffic drifted up from Marylebone Road to tell me it was time to get up, I lay in bed unable to sleep. And from my jumbled thoughts of anger and despair suddenly emerged, like a shooting star in a clear moonless sky, the precise concept of my new purpose in life:

No way was I going to let Andrew die.

I would devote myself to saving his life. And to helping him to save his own life.

I sprang out of bed. It would be a goal to strive for every minute of every day.

There was not a moment to be lost.

- 0 -

Colin took Andrew for X-rays in Harley Street at ten o'clock.

From Andrew's diary:

> *On arrival back at the flat I was in absolute agony. Mind you, at least it wasn't as bad as last night. I woke at four this morning in the worst pain I've ever had. I phoned Laura. I don't know what to do about Laura. I really am in love with her but somehow I don't think her feelings are the same for me. I'll go spare if she tells me where to*

87

go.

While they were out I had a phone call out of the blue from a woman who introduced herself as Janet Grayson. She told me they had heard about Andrew's illness from a mutual friend, and wanted to help us in any way they could.

I was moved by the warmth and sincerity of Janet Grayson's offer. I was also puzzled, but not for long. A year ago, she told me, their only son Paul had the same illness.

Osteosarcoma.

The Graysons gave us all a great deal of advice and support. Generously they passed on all their knowledge, though Paul had been treated by a different medical team.

This unique bond created a mutual empathy between the two boys, and Andrew gained much encouragement through his friendship with Paul.

In 1984 there were no cancer support groups like there are now. And no teenage support groups. Andrew was on his own. We were on our own, so the help we received from Philip and Jo Rodin, and from the Graysons was like gold dust. Now, many years later, we have the wonderful Teenage Cancer Trust, we have CLIC Sargent who look after children up to the age of twenty-four with cancer, and of course the Bone Cancer Research Trust who give support for young people with primary bone cancer.

Unfortunately Paul had a set-back just after he first met Andrew, and had to have chemotherapy and surgery to remove a tumour from his lung. Jo Rodin was afraid Andrew would think the same thing might happen to him, and warned against too much contact with Paul. I thought she was making a fuss about nothing but found out later that Andrew did indeed imagine that he too might develop metastases in his lungs, and suffered many agonies of doubt.

The vital difference in Paul's treatment was that he had no chemotherapy until after the operation to remove the tumour and insert the prosthesis. Poor ill-fated Terry Fox who ran one-legged across Canada to raise funds for cancer research had also had chemotherapy only after his amputation. But Andrew would have chemotherapy *before* the surgery. This newly developed difference had to be explained to Andrew when Paul was subsequently not well.

Paul phoned Andrew frequently during the week before the start of his treatment. When he came up to London one evening to meet Andrew for the first time, we could all see that he was a shining example of the potential success of the knee replacement surgery. He walked with only a very slight limp, hardly noticeable unless you were looking for it.

He vividly described the operation and his recovery. If he did depict the chemotherapy rather too luridly, this didn't seem to worry Andrew unduly. Knowing Paul made him feel he was not alone.

"He seems a very nice young man," I said, after Paul left.

"He is. And his leg is fantastic. Like a real leg. That's just what mine will be like. It's great. And you know what, Mum?"

"No, darling. What?"

"He's alive."

- 0 -

Next day there was a London Transport strike. Not one bus or underground train was running. I lay in bed listening to the earlier than usual roar of traffic floating up to the sixth floor from Marylebone Road, and thought what an unreal world we were living in now. How different all this was from our gloriously untroubled existence in the wide open spaces of Zambia, with our perfect weather, our relaxed social life, our games of golf, our swimming pools, our game parks. A paradise I had once thought would last forever.

Or had all that been the unreal world?

Was this noisy chaos really how the so-called civilised world was meant to be? A beautiful city, steeped in art and history, with its peaceful parks and graceful streets and elegant buildings engulfed by a never ending sea of traffic and noise and pollution?

I did not know. I clamped my hands over my ears and screwed up my eyes until I saw fiery whorls pulsing in and out of a blanket of purple velvet. The only thing I did know right now was that I must look after Andrew. I must love him and nurture him.

I must save his life.

- 0 -

I watched in horror the taxis crawl by in their hundreds, many with only one passenger. I waved and shouted but they all ignored me.

I glanced at my watch. I looked down at my useless feet. They were still painful but I could not afford to wait a moment longer.

Clutching the precious bottle in my hand I started walking.

I knew the way well, but did I know the best way to walk? I wasn't sure. I would just have to let instinct guide me.

Soon I realised it was much further than I thought and time was not on my side. The life of the sperm was limited. If I didn't get there in time I'd be killing part of Andrew.

I began to run. Razor blades tore at my feet and sent pain shooting up my legs. After five minutes I almost gave up.

This was a vital errand. One which might make the difference between having a grandchild and not having a grandchild; but it was not just that. As I ran I knew that not only was my new purpose in life to make sure that Andrew did not die, but there was nothing in this world that I would not do for him.

Then something strange happened.

The faster I ran the less pain I felt, until I realised I had no pain at all!

And suddenly I saw it. The Middlesex Hospital. Rising like a heavenly Mount Olympus to my distraught eyes. Hot, breathless, purple in the face and pleased as Punch, I handed over the bottle and took the new one from the technician. As I trudged slowly back from the hospital, every step like walking on a bed of nails now that nature's anaesthetic had worn off, my thoughts began to crystallize.

It was my fault that Andrew was suffering from this dreadful disease.

Why?

It must be. Somehow, somewhere, I must have done something wrong, or omitted to do something right. How else could he have got it? The doctors had told us that nobody knew what caused it, but isn't a mother responsible for her child's well-being? She has created him, fed him, cared for him, taught him. So it had to be something that I had done wrong.

I went over and over the pregnancy I'd been so thrilled to have at last achieved. Had I been too old to bear a child? Played too much golf? Gone to too many parties? Eaten the wrong foods? Stopped smoking too late?

I remembered my mother's words. "Sheila dear, you do too much. You must rest."

With at least another half a mile to walk and my feet unbearably painful, I stopped at a small café for a cup of coffee. As I sat on the hard red plastic chair I suddenly remembered Susie.

I had kicked Susie!

According to the doctor's calculation I still had three weeks to go. It was the middle of the night. I was terribly tired but couldn't sleep because Susie was barking her head off. Holding my enormous stomach with one hand I felt my way to the kitchen and told her to shut up. Ignoring her wagging tail and the delight in her soft brown eyes at seeing me, I told her again and again and again, but still she barked.

And then I kicked her. Lovely gentle adoring faithful Susie who I adored and had named Susan for the daughter I never had – unbelievably I kicked her.

As I crawled guiltily back into bed the waters broke, flooding me and the bedclothes with a gush of hot amniotic fluid. Andrew was born thirty-six hours later. Three weeks early. My other two had been three weeks late. It was the longest, most complicated, most painful birth of the three.

Could it have been that?

Or could it have been the car accident at the roundabout in Kitwe, when the car in front of me suddenly stopped when he had right of way? With a grinding of metal and a shattering of glass my little white Ford Popular had ploughed into him. I had the steering wheel to hold on to but Andrew was thrown into the dash-board, his right leg smashing into the gear lever with a sickening thud.

Oh my God ...

With the uncovered guilt gnawing at every atom of my being I limped back to the flat and that night I had a strange and terrible dream. It was so real that I had no idea that it was a dream. I wanted it to be a dream. Oh, how I willed it to be a dream, but even when I was fully awake I was convinced it had actually happened.

For weeks I fought to suppress the dream. Night and day the images invaded my thoughts, confronting me with their stark horror.

But instead of becoming less horrific each day, the images grew with savage force. I was punished with their increasing intensity. They lived with me constantly. The hunting knife became a double-edged sword, needle sharp and spiny, sharper than a butcher's knife, bloodier than a surgeon's. The laughter blasted through my head like the shrill of a dentist's drill, shrieking and jangling and clattering and reverberating as it grew louder and fiercer and more accusing. And it seemed that on those nights when I strove the hardest to avoid the dream it would visit me in its most violent form.

Each time it returned it strengthened my resolve: I must live with my guilt, but somehow I must make it up to Andrew.

He must live.

- 0 -

"We can't go on staying in this expensive flat," Colin said one morning at breakfast. He was studying the latest bank balance which had gone down drastically in the last few weeks. "Soon there will be nothing left."

Janet Grayson was full of advice about our proposed new abode. "It must be on the ground floor or have a reliable lift. It must have a walk-in shower. After Paul's operation it was ages before he could manage stairs or get in and out of the bath. And don't forget that chemotherapy destroys the white blood cells. It leaves the body with no resistance so it must be something very clean and well maintained."

We began the search, but the rents were all enormous. Even higher than we were paying now.

Then I had a brainwave.

Zach. My old childhood friend from Cape Town. A director of the richest and most powerful company in South Africa, with strong connections in London. I telephoned their London office for his Johannesburg number. The secretary offered to make the call for me. Next day she phoned back. "Dr de Beer will fix something up and let you know soon," she said.

Fantastic! I could hardly believe our luck.

- 0 -

Colin had finally got all the figures together and there was no way the medical insurance companies and our own available funds would cover all the medical expenses. After hours of calculations and straight down-to-earth logistics, he made the big decision:

92

"Andrew will have to be treated under the NHS. Either that or we'll become hopelessly in debt"

"Philip and Jo will be pleased," I said, nodding my agreement.

Colin tried all day to get hold of Mr Adanar and eventually left a message with his secretary. When Mr Adanar phoned back that evening he said that changing to the NHS meant performing the operation at the teaching hospital where he practised in his NHS capacity, instead of at the private hospital where he'd done Andrew's biopsy. "But this will cause insoluble complications," he explained, "because Dr Jelliffe is based at The Middlesex Hospital. It'll be impossible to combine the NHS treatment at two different hospitals, so I've asked Mr Sweetnam, who is also based at The Middlesex, to take over the surgical treatment. Mr Sweetnam has agreed."

Oh wow! This was amazing news.

Colin thanked Mr Adanar for everything he had done, then phoned Philip and Jo to tell them. They were delighted.

It was exactly what they'd been angling for.

"Frankly," Philip said, "we were dismayed that you could even contemplate having such costly treatment done privately, when we told you it could be carried out far more safely and efficiently within the National Health Service which has all the available facilities. And now," he added gleefully, "you will be having the best surgeon for the job."

That night Andrew went to see Laura, to tell her the good news.

What a fantastic evening with Laura. That certainly was something I had not expected at all. I hardly had any sleep but God was it worth it! We came back to Baker Street then went to Muswells for lunch. It's really annoying though. Laura will not let me pay for anything. I'll have to take her out some time for a really first class meal. I've come to the conclusion once again that I do love Laura. I know I've said before much the same thing about other girls but this is different. She's the most loving, kind, warm-hearted friend I know.

- 0 -

As the start of Andrew's treatment drew uncomfortably close, an air of irritability and edginess had begun to permeate the atmosphere. With all the X-rays and tests completed it seemed we were beginning to get on each other's nerves and were unconsciously seeking the company of friends outside the family for some light relief. One day, Andrew, quite at home on his crutches now, took Laura to a nearby restaurant before she went on afternoon shift; Colin had lunch in the City with his old university friend, Brian Baverstock, and I met Dave and Peggy at Martha's Wine Bar for a salad.

I was the first one home. Just after I arrived there was a phone call from the personnel manager of the Diamond Trading Company in Holborn telling me that Zach de Beer had been in touch with them.

"We have a ground floor flat you could move into on the ninth of April," he said.

Oblivious of my crippled feet I danced around the room, pirouetting and leaping from one end of the carpet to the other.

"Oh Zach! Thank you thank you thank you!" I yelled as I waited to tell the others.

- 0 -

Andrew had straight shiny golden blond hair, thick and healthy. He wanted it cut before going into hospital on Monday, so on Saturday morning we found a nice barber in Marylebone Road and asked for 'the works'.

The barber remarked on the fine quality of the hair. What a pity, I thought sadly, to have such a super cut and blow-dry when Dr Jelliffe had warned it could soon all fall out.

With the school term just ended, James, one of Andrew's special best friends, arrived to take him out for lunch. With a lump in my throat I watched from the window of our sixth floor flat. Watched the strong healthy James guide Andrew on his crutches over busy Marylebone Road. Watched them disappear slowly down the street towards McDonald's.

"It's not fair!" I shouted to the walls.

Then I took a deep breath. Don't be ridiculous, I told myself. You must not give way to these feelings of despair. Jo said you must keep strong and prop up the rest of the family. How can you give in now?

When Andrew came back it was good to see him looking so happy. He had missed James and his other two special friends, Simon and

94

Stuart, who had been too busy with mock A-levels to visit him often. Andrew felt the isolation of being suddenly cut off from his closest friends and it was one of the tragedies of the illness that he would miss not only his A-level exams but the last six months of his school career.

- 0 -

It was noon on Sunday. Only one day to go. Peter had come down for the day and Jo had invited us all for lunch.

Gliding through the deserted streets in Philip's automatic Mercedes, past the majestic old buildings of the City, the Old Bailey, the Bank of England, St Paul's; over the swiftly flowing Thames and past the green oasis of Blackheath common to their elegant townhouse in a quiet leafy square, I could not help thinking how lucky we were to have met the Rodins on that idyllic deserted beach in Menorca.

We talked and talked and talked. We even managed a few laughs. We were all over-conscious of what tomorrow had in store for Andrew, but miraculously he stayed cheerful. Somehow he succeeded in putting us all at ease as though he did not want to be responsible for our unhappiness.

- 0 -

"Dad, come and sit on my suitcase, please."

Colin sat on one end and I sat on the other.

"Good heavens, Andrew! What have you got in here?"

He opened the case and started unpacking it in order to re-pack it properly. On top were three pairs of new shorty-pyjamas and the shiny new combination TV-radio-cassette recorder we had bought in Marylebone Road on Saturday. Underneath were piles of books.

Colin started hauling them out. "What do you want all these for, son?"

"They're my English A-level set books. Put them back, Dad. I need them."

Colin re-stacked them neatly and managed to close the suitcase. Andrew got into bed and we tucked him in like a baby.

"I wonder what it'll be like," he said wistfully, and I knew then for sure that he was scared.

95

I pushed back the shiny golden hair that had fallen over his forehead. I swallowed hard. "It'll be ... fine," I said.

He looked up and caught my hand, then reached for Colin's too.

"You mustn't worry, you two," he said with a little smile that pursed his lips together and turned up the corners of his mouth. "I'll be okay."

As we tiptoed out I rammed my knuckles against my mouth.

My heart ached for him. He was trying so hard to be brave.

Chapter Nine

From the back seat of the black London taxi the Monday morning traffic looked perfectly normal. The people thronging the West End streets looked perfectly normal. But once we drove into the forecourt of The Middlesex Hospital nothing was perfectly normal any more.

For this was the start of a period of Andrew's life when he would suffer more than any eighteen year old should ever have to suffer. A period when the future – if there were to be a future – was a large black bottomless void, totally unknown.

We walked in and took our seats on hard metal chairs placed in rows along one side of the high-ceilinged entrance hall, feeling like convicted prisoners awaiting their verdicts.

After fifteen minutes Andrew's name was called. At the desk a plastic-coated bracelet was attached to his wrist. He was number 324317.

Greenhow Ward was on the third floor, far left hand side of the building, in the area of the hospital allocated to cancer patients. With its bare scrubbed floors and twelve basic beds it had none of the luxury of the private hospital. No fancy control panels to zoom the beds up and down, no remote controls for light switches, radios or television sets. No pictures on the walls, no wall-to-wall carpets.

But right inside the ward, in full view of all the beds, was the nurses' station.

I liked that.

On the white painted bedside table of bed number twelve stood a jug of water and a plastic glass. Sister disapproved when we moved these aside to install Andrew's shiny new television set.

"You can keep it this time, Andrew, but you must not bring it in future." She was tiny but there was great authority in her voice.

After the usual blood pressure, pulse, temperature and urine tests, came the blood test. Not as bad as the one at the private hospital, since Andrew knew now what to expect, but it was never going to be easy because the needle phobia caused the veins to shrink and almost disappear, making it practically impossible to insert the needle without much painful probing.

I often wonder if the medical staff was aware that this was a deep-down fear, not just some squeamish little thing in the mind of a spoilt child. Living in a tropical African country, Andrew was subjected from an early age to frequent jabs for cholera and smallpox, sometimes every few months for cholera. During epidemics, auxiliary Red Cross nurses often carried out mass inoculations at schools, and once when he was only five years old he was frightened by one of these well-meaning helpers who came at him with her needle like the villain in one of his *Spider Man* comics. When he went away a year later to Whitestone School in Bulawayo, and the whole school had to stand in line outside the sanatorium every three months for their cholera jabs, Andrew was thrown into a panic by the memory of the over-eager Red Cross nurse. Terrified, he would cringe and try to run away.

- 0 -

At first the atmosphere in the ward seemed a bit depressing, but the mostly elderly men in the other eleven beds were very pleasant and soon Andrew was chatting to them all. After a couple of hours, when we thought he was well settled, Colin and I left the hospital to go and have some lunch.

This was a big mistake.

It never occurred to us that we should not have left him alone. He was eighteen. Though still at school he was technically a man, but was he a child-man or an adult-man? He was in an adult ward because he was eighteen, but perhaps putting him with the older men was not the wisest thing to do. Today there are special teenage wards for these young men.

When the treatment was about to begin he became frightened. He tried phoning us at the flat but we were still out having lunch, so he phoned Jenny and luckily she was at home.

I was utterly dismayed when we got back and found a great commotion going on behind closed screens: Jenny on one side holding his hand, several nurses in attendance, and Dr Annabel Brown desperately trying to insert the needle in his vein.

I was furious. Why hadn't we been told what was going to happen and when it would happen? After weeks of our continued support he suddenly found himself on his own and panicked. Just when we were needed we weren't there.

"I want this all to go away," Andrew said, tossing his head from side to side, his lips quivering. "This isn't really happening. Is it, Mum?"

Later we found out the sequence of events for each treatment. First the blood and urine tests to determine the blood count and kidney function. Then a blood transfusion, but only if the count is too low. Next, a twenty-four hour saline drip. This promotes the flow of water through the kidneys, protecting them from the toxic effects of the drugs which can cause kidney failure. It also prepares the system for the vicious onslaught of heavy metals in the chemotherapy 'cocktail' specially concocted for osteosarcoma.

And then finally the three-day programme of chemotherapy, preceded in each case by the pre-medication and the ice-cap. Most of the drugs are delivered intravenously, some orally, with small doses of cannabis thrown in to help induce a state of euphoria. Anti-memory drugs are added in the hope that they will blot out the worst horrors of the treatment, otherwise – if he is one of the unlucky ones who are badly affected by the chemo – the patient might never agree to have the next session. Usually this works but sometimes it doesn't. Sometimes it is so ghastly that the patient remembers vividly.

We were sure this would never happen to Andrew.

On this first occasion though, it was all new. Although Paul had told Andrew how nasty it was, clearly you had to experience it to understand the agonies involved. Before it started Andrew's one thought had been, *this is going to cure me*. He'd been apprehensive, a bit scared, but not really afraid. Now he fought against every step, not accepting any part of it graciously.

Jo Rodin said this rebellion was a good thing.

"People like Andrew," she said when I phoned her, "who question every move and complain bitterly about the pain and discomfort, will probably recover well." These words were not only comforting but thought provoking too. Was this fighting spirit necessary, I wondered, to combat the disease?

Horrified, we looked on. No amount of pre-medication – not the cannabis, valium, or any other drug they gave him – calmed him down.

"What are they doing to me, Mum? What's going on?"

I wished I could help. I wished with all my heart that I could go through it for him.

After three attempts to get the drip up Dr Annabel was forced to give him more valium. An hour later when he was knocked right out, she succeeded in getting the needle into his right hand. Even then it was not easy as the veins had almost disappeared.

- 0 -

The following morning before we went to the hospital a complete stranger phoned. He had heard about Andrew from an acquaintance of ours and said he wanted to help. He'd also had cancer, he told me, though not osteosarcoma. His leg had been amputated but he managed very well now, riding a bicycle and carrying on his job as a dentist. "Please tell Andrew never to give up," he said, with so much empathy in his voice that it was hard to believe we had never met. I put down the phone with a warm feeling inside me.

Andrew was not very keen on the hospital food so Colin made him his favourite bacon and tomato sandwich for his lunch. When we arrived back we found him bright and cheerful, hopping all over the ward on one leg, chatting to the other patients, using the drip stand as a crutch.

He was well aware of how ill all the other patients were, but had developed a particular rapport with a man of about thirty-five with cancer of the liver. As he ate his bacon sandwich he told us he'd just had a long chat with this man.

"The doctors came in to see him and I could see he was very upset," Andrew told us. "When they left I went over to talk to him. Oh, Mum. They'd told him there was nothing more they could do for him. That he had only a few more months to live. I tried to comfort him but he's so worried about his wife and his two little girls ..."

- 0 -

That night I felt guilty when we set off for the Royal Albert Hall to see John Curry's 'Symphony on Ice'. There was so much suffering around me and I was convinced it would be impossible to enjoy the evening.

But I was wrong. Marvelling at the adaptability of this wondrous building with its crimson seats, the gilded arches, the Victorian ornamentation, the grand circular sweep of the auditorium and now the sheet of glittering ice, I was swept away on a wave of euphoria at the grace and beauty of the show. It occurred to me afterwards that incongruously my intense enjoyment of the skating had somehow been heightened by my intense sadness.

- 0 -

On Wednesday morning Colin Junior phoned from Zambia with a long list of get-well wishes from friends over there. We passed these on to Andrew just as he was being started on a new drip. This time it was sodium bicarbonate to counteract the acidity of the chemo drugs that were due to be injected in a few hours' time.

The little ward Sister, not more than four feet eleven, with her cute upturned nose and her big green eyes so full of tenderness and concern, came to Andrew's bedside and knelt down next to him with a gruesome looking object on a tray.

Andrew looked at it sideways. "Crumbs," he said. "What's *that*?"

"It's an ice-cap, Andrew. We'll put it on your head half an hour before the chemo drugs are injected and I'd like you to hold it now, so you can feel how heavy it is."

Andrew took it gingerly, turned it over and handed it back, wondering what all the fuss was about. It was in its unfrozen state, so he did not appreciate what it would be like when ice cold.

"Chemo drugs kill all fast-growing cells, Andrew, so one of the side effects is loss of hair," she said soberly. "The ice-cap will stop the drug-laden blood from flowing to the roots of your hair, so, if it works, you won't lose it all."

She smiled and ran her fingers through the golden blond hair lying tousled on his forehead. "Don't worry, Andrew. We'll give you a pre-med one hour before. This'll make you so sleepy you won't even be aware of the ice-cap."

But the pre-med did not make Andrew sleepy. Nor did it make him drowsy or calm. Or even slightly unaware of the ice-cap.

"No! Take it away!" he yelled, his shoulders hunching and his neck twisting this way and that as they tried to put the cold, hard, heavy gadget on his head. Just as they got it on he yanked it off again, but at last, in spite of his wild protestations, they succeeded.

Half an hour later the slender, blonde Dr Annabel Brown injected the chemotherapy drugs into the drip. Adriamycin and Cisplatin, a pinky red mixture which to my surprise appeared to cause acute pain

101

as it entered Andrew's body. Then, to protect the drugs from the action of light, they popped a brown paper bag over the infusion as it continued its menacing drip drip drip ...

I sat close to Andrew, holding his hand until eventually he dropped off to sleep. Incredulously I looked at the array of needles and tubes and bottles, and the brown paper bag that seemed to be a grim reminder of a patient undergoing chemotherapy treatment.

Colin glanced at me and we shook our heads. I looked down at the pale sheen of Andrew's now peaceful face. Was all this going to make him live, I wondered.

Slowly I extracted my hand from his. As we tiptoed out past the rows of silent beds, we found Jo Rodin and Andrew's cousin Timothy waiting to take us for a drink at The Swan, just across the road.

English pubs are unique. With their panelled walls and subdued lights they offer to the weary traveller a haven of convenience and comfort and company.

"I don't see how that awful looking gunge they injected into Andrew is supposed to cure him," I said when Colin had brought our drinks over from the bar. "I just don't understand it."

We were always learning from Jo and this was no exception. As we sipped our drinks she explained to us the mysteries of chemotherapy. About how in some way the aggressive drugs interfere with the cell cycle, attacking the DNA of the rapidly dividing malignant cells.

"It stops them from multiplying," she said. "Melts them away so that the tumour actually shrinks."

That night the Graysons visited us at the flat. They had been to visit Paul who was then also in hospital having chemo for the tumour in his lung. It helped so much to talk. We learned a great deal from their frank discussion and the more we learned the less afraid we became.

- 0 -

Dr Annabel was discovering how much it took to knock Andrew right out, and on Thursday things went far more smoothly. He was asleep or almost asleep most of the day, and whenever he was awake I sat on the bed and held his hand.

Later in the afternoon he had three other visitors.

First Laura.

Although he was asleep I had the feeling he knew she was there.

102

She seemed to give him a sense of security. I could see that she was very special to him. She was his girlfriend. She was his lover.

Young James from Bradfield College was next, and then Jenny. The three of them sat huddled together next to the bed, talking in hushed whispers while Andrew slept.

It was unfortunate that he was one of the few who Dr Jelliffe had said reacted very badly to the drugs. Although fairly well knocked out for the rest of the week, he vomited frequently and suffered terrible headaches. Some people got away with just vague feelings of nausea. Others could not tolerate the fierce assault of the chemicals on the lining of the stomach and intestines.

Dr Annabel Brown was conscientious, gentle and understanding. Andrew was steadily gaining confidence in her but he still did not take lightly to any of it.

Each afternoon followed the same routine: the pre-med, the ice-cap, the chemo injection, with the drip shrouded in the brown paper bag hanging ominously over him.

More than anything else he hated the ice-cap. He often tried to take it off but in his doped condition could never quite manage it, though once he inveigled a nurse to take it off after only half an hour because he couldn't stand the pain.

I hated it too. I had to sit there and watch them putting this ill-fitting monstrosity on his head. I had to watch him writhe in agony. Watch the tears run down his cheeks. One small block of ice held against my skin is excruciatingly painful so I shuddered to think what this huge evil looking object would feel like.

Suspecting that it wasn't very well designed because of its clumsy, square shape when frozen, I had a good look at it and could see that it was being badly utilized because it only had contact with about fifty percent of the head. This was because it consisted of flat, rectangular segments which could only have fitted someone with a square head.

I cornered one of the nurses. "Wouldn't it be more effective if it were frozen more or less to the shape of a head?" I asked, as politely as I could. It's soft and pliable when unfrozen, so couldn't you mould it onto something round?"

But they continued to freeze it flat. Andrew grew to hate it more and more. Coming as a prelude to the chemo drugs, it epitomised for him the whole ghastly experience. He got sick every time it was put on his head. It became a symbolic reminder of the forthcoming invasion of toxic drugs and he even got sick when he saw them approaching him with the ice-cap on a tray. He was never reconciled to it, right up to the end when they were finally forced to abandon it. It was a complete waste of time anyway, because eventually every single hair fell out of Andrew's head and his body.

- 0 -

In spite of everything, Andrew remained relatively cheerful. He was under no illusion. He knew he'd had a fantastic reprieve: his leg was going to be saved; he was going to remain whole; the girls would still love him.

Though Colin and I were both frantic with worry, we too were very relieved that Andrew would not lose his leg. But suddenly – out of the blue – this security was threatened.

Chapter Ten

It is lunch time and we are back at the flat having a quick bite to eat when the phone rings.

It's the little Sister from Greenhow Ward.

"Will you please come to the hospital," she says.

Her usually soft, gentle voice is tinged with urgency and my insides do a U-turn as I wonder what she wants.

"Dr Jelliffe would like to see you right away."

My heart starts pounding as we tear out of the flat and grab the first taxi we see.

"Why do you think he wants to see us?" Col's pale blue eyes are drawn together in a frown, his voice almost a whisper.

I shake my head, not even daring to guess.

We are ushered into the consulting room. Dr Jelliffe invites us to sit down. His mouth has tightened into a hard line that we have not seen before.

"I feel I must tell you —"

I hold my breath. His voice is calm, level and kind so it can't be anything too bad ...

"That although all preparations are being made to save Andrew's leg —"

My pulse quickens ...

"It may be necessary to amputate it."

My thoughts leap to Andrew ...

"Not even the nuclear scan, let alone all the other X-rays Andrew will have before the surgery, will tell us whether or not the precious tendons and arteries are being affected by the cancer."

The consulting room is small, the chairs hard, the walls cream and unadorned. Outside in the passage there are footsteps and voices and beyond the window the blaring blasting tumult of the city. But for me there is only Dr Jelliffe's face. And his kind eyes. And his words piercing the air like daggers ripping through my body.

"For the operation to be a success the first priority is to get the

105

tumour away, so it must be removed in its entirety. But if too much normal tissue has to be removed in the process, like blood vessels, arteries, muscle and tendons needed to support the leg, then there would be problems with the prosthesis, and we would not be able to go ahead."

He pauses.

He looks first at my face and then at Colin's. He speaks in layman's terms, making it easy for us to understand. But now, perhaps because we have not said a single word, I guess he doesn't know if we have taken anything in and he seems uncertain of how to carry on.

"Nobody knows yet what will happen. The surgeons will not be able to tell until they open up the leg in June, whether there is enough healthy tissue left to enable them to complete the planned reconstruction with the metal prosthesis Professor Scales is designing to replace the diseased bones. Because each case is different we don't even have statistics to help us make a calculated guess."

I suddenly wonder why it is Dr Jelliffe, the physician, telling us this, and not Mr Sweetnam, the surgeon. Then I remember that the physician is the *healer*; the one concerned with the total person; with his emotions; with the quality of his future life. Mr Sweetnam is saving Andrew's leg, but Dr Jelliffe is saving Andrew's life, regardless of the fate of the leg.

I see a muscle twitch in Colin's sheet-white cheek but still he says nothing. For once I too am mute. I must pull myself together. I have a feeling I can cope with this news better than Colin can. As a man he is automatically putting himself in Andrew's place; he will know how devastating it would be to suddenly be a one-legged man. I on the other hand must think as a mother. Right. They are going to save my son's life whichever way they can and if that means chopping off his leg to do it then that's okay with me.

Just as long as he lives.

We remain silent, so Dr Jelliffe carries on. He senses our anguish. "However," he says gently, "it's most important that Andrew should not be told yet about the possibility of amputation. This news would distress him and affect his tolerance of the chemotherapy drugs. It would be best not to tell anybody else either, in case it leaked to Andrew."

This makes sense but worries me. It's never easy to deceive members of a close-knit family who've been taught to be honest and open with each other; they can recognise all too easily when something is being held back, leading to distrust and fear and a reciprocal lack of honesty. After Mr Adanar's final diagnosis Andrew and I were told separately, then together, so that Andrew would know that I knew that he knew too; but now it is different. Now Andrew has embarked upon a course of treatment which could temporarily reduce his normal powers of mental endurance to a low level. First and foremost it is important to protect him. I understand this only too well.

"We'll watch carefully for a suitable moment to tell him," Dr Jelliffe says as he sees us to the door. "A moment when we consider he is able to take it."

Like two victims of an earthquake stumbling dazed from the rubble, we return to Greenhow Ward.

With glazed eyes Andrew looks from one of us to the other.

"What's up with you two?" he asks, half asleep but clearly sensing that something is amiss.

"Nothing," Colin says, as we both try to disguise our shock. "We were just having a little chat with Dr Jelliffe."

He looks at us askance but probes no further. I guess this is not because he is afraid of what he might hear, but because he knows that whatever it is, it might hurt us to have to tell him. As we leave the ward I turn to wave, but already he is fast asleep. He will eventually be told, but for the moment this added torment will not be included in his ordeal.

- 0 -

Naively expecting to feel well immediately the treatment ended on Friday afternoon, Andrew had been planning a weekend outing with Laura; but this was not to be. He finally left his hospital bed on Saturday afternoon and moved straight into his bed at the flat. When friends arrived for the home-coming supper we'd organised, he made a gallant attempt to join us at the table, but couldn't eat a thing.

"It's like a monstrous hangover," he said when I helped him back to bed.

Next morning he seemed much brighter. He got up and showered and even made his bed like a good boarding school boy, but half an hour later he was sick again. I sat with him on his bed, holding his hand, feeling inadequate in my inability to help him.

107

A dog-eared copy of TS Eliot's poems lay open on the pillow. He picked it up and read aloud two lines from *The Love Song of J Alfred Prufrock*.

"And would it have been worth it, after all,
Would it have been worth while ..."

He closed the book and we looked deep into each other's eyes. Eventually, unable to speak, I nodded. Slowly he nodded back.

Eliot had spoken for him.

"Is it, Mum ...?" he said with a sudden frown. "Is it really all worth it?"

"Yes, darling, of course it's worth it. Because you are going to get well."

He retched again and I held him until the spasms subsided. "This is awful for you, I know, but you have to put up with it. When it's all over you'll know it was worth while."

"You don't know just how awful it is, Mum."

No. I did not know. And neither was I able to tell him that with each bolt of pain, each spasm of nausea, each tremor of fear, I was there with him, although I think perhaps he guessed I was.

Throughout the day, each time he vomited and I held his shivering body, I told myself it was all going to be worth while.

- 0 -

We had arranged to move to our new flat at the Diamond Trading Company on Monday morning. Andrew was due for a CT scan in the afternoon, but I was alarmed when I woke up at six o'clock to yet more sounds of vomiting.

He was sitting up in bed with the basin in front of him. His hair stood up in spikes. Perspiration ran down his pallid face.

"I feel awful, Mum, and I've got this ringing in my ears." He clamped his hands over his ears. "It's driving me mad and I can't sleep. Oh, I wish I could sleep."

I sponged his face with a wet cloth then hurried to the kitchen to squeeze a couple of oranges and puree some apple. I felt so helpless. I didn't know what to do. He looked so weak so the least I could do was make sure he had something to eat.

Even that didn't stay down, so while Colin threw everything into suitcases and cardboard boxes to move to the new flat, I took Andrew back to the hospital.

As we walked into Greenhow Ward Dr Annabel Brown took one look at Andrew's white face and hurried towards us. She looked tired, as though she'd been up all night, and with her tall slender figure shrouded in a crisp white coat and her long blonde hair scraped back in a bun, one might almost not have noticed what an attractive young woman she was.

But attractive was the least of Dr Annabel's virtues. With a look of genuine concern on her face she helped Andrew to a chair, then checked his pulse, temperature and blood pressure.

"You must have at least two litres of fluid a day," she told him. "The ringing in your ears is caused by lack of body fluids due to the chemo drugs and all the vomiting. But if you still feel sick tomorrow you'll have to come back into hospital. I'll make sure there's a bed for you, Andrew."

I wished I had known about this fluid thing sooner, but nobody had told me.

It was now almost time for his chest X-ray and CT scan. Andrew was curious about the procedure so Dr Annabel explained that CT is short for Computerised Tomography. She didn't underestimate Andrew's intelligence so did not mince her words.

"The CT Scanner is cleverer than an ordinary X-ray machine," she told him, "because it can detect subtle changes in the tissues of the body, depending on the water content of each area. You can see the true size of tumours and locate sites of spread."

Andrew blinked.

"You'll have to lie on a table for about forty-five minutes while a huge revolving disc moves up and down shooting X-rays from different angles. This is linked to a computer which calculates the tissue density at different sites, producing pictures of slices through the body based on their differing water content."

- 0 -

He had a grin on his face when he came out. "I could actually see those pictures on the screen, Mum. It was hard to realise it was me. I didn't know what I was looking at but I could see that there was something mighty wrong."

To illustrate this he drew pictures of the 'slices' he remembered.

109

One from his left leg. One from the right. The circle he drew to represent the right leg was far larger than for the left, and the central area depicting the bone was twice as big and much darker.

He had drawn the tumour.

- 0 -

Our new home – appropriately called St. Andrew's House – was behind the Diamond Trading Building in Charterhouse Street on the western border of the old 'City' of London. With its white wrought iron balconies it resembled an old Kimberley building from the diamond rush days in South Africa, and to the three of us was a haven of peace after the hustle and bustle of Marylebone Road.

Flat number three was spacious and comfortable. By the time Andrew and I arrived, Colin had done wonders and already it looked like home.

The building faces a large courtyard formed by the right angle of the two wings of the Diamond Building, one in wide, elegant Charterhouse Street, the other teetering on narrow, one-way Saffron Hill. On the map of Dickens' London, displayed on the wall of the Bleeding Heart restaurant just around the corner, it occupied the very spot of Fagin's den, described by Dickens as a 'place of filth and evil'. Now, ironically, it is the spot where almost every diamond in the world is either bought or sold – the world's largest single source of rough diamonds – and enjoys the best security in the capital!

Next morning Andrew still felt dreadful. He forced down yet another glass of water and at last began to improve. Colin took him to the Royal Orthopaedic Hospital where more X-rays and measurements were taken for the artificial knee and tibia to be constructed by Professor Scales, Professor of Biomedical Engineering, who some years earlier pioneered the design and construction of the replacement prostheses to be used by Mr Sweetnam in his revolutionary new treatment of osteosarcoma.

A few days later Colin flew back to Zambia.

With my heart breaking I watched father and son cling to each other, both with strained smiles and red-rimmed eyes. How devoted they are, I thought. More devoted than ever before. How precious is love. Especially when it is threatened.

"Come back soon, Dad," Andrew said.

110

Now on our own Andrew and I began to establish a new relationship: an understanding and closeness which ironically could never have evolved if Andrew had not been critically ill.

Yet it was not all plain sailing.

A few days after Colin left, Andrew was sitting in front of the TV with a face like thunder. I put my arms around him to comfort him.

"Leave me alone!" he said, scowling and turning away.

I withdrew, too stunned to say anything. I went into the kitchen and put the kettle on, then sat at the table drinking a cup of my favourite, comforting Rooibos tea. A few minutes later he suddenly appeared behind me. Encircling me with his arms he held me tight, resting his cheek against my head.

He was sobbing.

"I didn't mean to hurt you, Mum. I'm so sorry. I love you."

It was quite uncanny the way Jo had predicted the way he would behave. I would say to myself, "Well, that's what Jo said would happen and there you are, it is happening. It's quite natural and it will pass."

Not that this knowledge prevented me being hurt by the shocks and knocks he dealt to me during those first difficult weeks, but I understood, therefore quickly adjusted. There was a 'give-and-take' between us which could not have developed if, in ignorance, I had reacted negatively to his displays of bitter temper, his moroseness, his petulant discontent, and his churlish ingratitude when I tried too hard to help him.

As his initial anger slowly abated, so was he less likely to vent his feelings on me. Gradually he began to accept the situation and was not so intensely preoccupied with thoughts of being disabled. I would smile quietly to myself when I observed how remarkably well he was adjusting for one so young. I began to recognise the strength of character so similar to that of my father who had remained cheerful all his life in spite of his crippling physical disabilities.

This acceptance did not mean that he now lay back and took it all resignedly. Oh no! Far from it. He still rebelled against the treatment he had to receive, but no longer imagined he had been singled out.

"I'm not the only one this has ever happened to, Mum. There are other teenagers in the same boat. Some far worse than me. I've got to fight it if I want to get better."

- 0 -

On Monday we had good news.

Dr Annabel phoned to say that the CT chest scan and X-rays were perfectly clear.

Oh what rejoicing!

This meant that there was no spread of the cancer to the lungs – the biggest fear in osteosarcoma. With a shiver down my spine I thought of what might have happened if Philip had not intervened.

Dr Annabel also gave Andrew the full programme planned for his treatment: two more chemo sessions, one at the end of April and the middle of May; admittance to Dressmakers Ward on the fourth of June; nuclear scan on the fifth, and the operation on the seventh. Another chemo session in June, two in July, with the treatment finally ending on the third of August.

Formidable. But at least Andrew now knew when it was all going to happen.

And when it would all be over.

"I'll write these dates in my diary," he said, then smiled. "That's great! It'll all be over just before Peter and Andrea's wedding."

I frowned. "Do you think you'll be well enough to go?"

"Course I will, Mum. I wouldn't miss it for anything."

I hoped he was right. Because if he could not go, how could I?

He saw the doubt in my eyes. "Just you wait. I bet you I'll even dance at Peter's wedding."

I put my arm around him.

"Of course you will," I said, and squeezed him tight.

- 0 -

Four of the girls from a school in Fleet who came regularly to the Bradfield College dances, arrived at the flat on Tuesday morning like a breath of spring air, complete with bunches of daffodils, laughter and love. Simon, one of Andrew's three best friends, came too and they all decided to go to *The Old Mitre*, a quaint little pub nearby. Hidden in a narrow alleyway between Hatton Garden and Ely Place, you approach it by a small hole in a wall which you miss if you walk too quickly.

112

Andrew liked the free and easy atmosphere and it became our 'local' when he was well enough to go out with friends.

I put the four enormous bunches of daffodils in a vase and thought, as I always do, what a happy colour yellow is.

"Take your crutches, Andrew," I said as they prepared to leave.

"I don't need them," he retorted, hating my intervention.

"Okay. Just take your stick."

"Mum! I don't need it!"

Biting my lip I watched them walk down the ramp, Andrew stubbornly and proudly and stupidly ignoring my nagging because he so badly wanted to be as normal as they all were.

That evening I stole a glance at the wistful expression in his sad, dark-rimmed eyes. The day had tired him out and for the first time ever I saw wrinkles on his pale, thin face.

Wrinkles! At eighteen.

He caught me looking at him. "I think I'll go to bed now, Mum."

And when I peeped in five minutes later he was asleep.

Yet each day the debilitating effects of the chemo were receding. So much so that he began to make plans to return to school for twelve days after his next treatment.

"But Andrew, have you forgotten how ill you were for the first week?"

"Mum. Stop fussing. I'll be fine."

Clearly the anti-memory drugs were working and there was nothing I could do to stop him.

"It's okay, Mum. My housemaster is arranging for me to have a big room downstairs, and he says I must only work on my English, otherwise I'll get too tired."

He came and sat next to me on the sofa and kissed my cheek. How could I say no? School was vitally important to him, and so were his friends.

Half an hour later he was phoning the master in charge of the school swimming team, making plans about helping to train the junior team during those twelve days.

I shook my head. I knew it was pointless to say anything.

- 0 -

I lie in bed reading. Andrew is unusually quiet. Normally I hear him

113

soon after he wakes up but this morning there is an ominous silence.

I get up quietly, a speciality of mine. I squeeze a couple of oranges and tiptoe to his room.

I open the door.

He is sitting up in bed, staring into space.

He turns his head slowly. His eyes frighten me. They are like fathomless pools. The more I look into them the more lacklustre they appear.

"Bad news, Mum."

He points to his pillow.

To a large tuft of hair, as dead looking as his eyes are.

He lifts his hand to his head and with a gentle tug plucks out another big handful.

I swallow hard. I had noticed about a week ago that his beautiful shiny blond hair had become dull. It had also changed to a dirty, muddy brownish colour which accentuated the red rims round his eyes and the ebony dark circles beneath them.

"I wouldn't worry, Andrew," I say gaily. "You have plenty of hair. You won't miss that little bit."

All morning he sits tugging at it. He phones Dr Annabel to tell her and she is very disappointed. She must be thinking what I am thinking – about the pain the useless ice-caps had caused.

To take his mind off it I take him to Leicester Square to see Clint Eastwood in *Sudden Impact*. He nudges me several times during the film.

"Mum! She's exactly like Dr Annabel!"

He's right. The leading lady has a tall willowy figure, long blonde hair, blue eyes and a smile that would knock any man flat. She looks exactly like Dr Annabel.

But this blonde is also a vicious killer.

He seems strangely morose for the rest of the day. He goes to bed early.

About midnight he wakes up screaming.

I rush into his room.

Dr Annabel is sawing off his leg.

- 0 -

The following night I had my dream again, and when I awoke I was

114

convinced I had not been asleep at all.

I got up early and made an extra effort to make Andrew's breakfast appetising. He was becoming alarmingly thin and I needed to build him up in readiness for the next chemotherapy treatment, which nobody so far was mentioning.

I knocked at the door and walked in with the tray. He was lying flat on his back staring into space. He pointed to the pillow.

"Look," he said.

Chunky tufts of hair covered his pillow, but this time it wasn't just one tuft. It looked like a whole head of hair and reminded me of my long-lashed Shirley Temple doll whose shiny ringlets had floated clean off her head when without my mother's knowledge I took her into the bath with me.

I put the tray down in front of him and with a nonchalant sweep I brushed the hair off the pillow into the waste paper basket.

"Why not try one of the wigs the NHS have offered you?" I suggested.

He scowled. "I wouldn't be seen dead in one of those."

I didn't blame him. They always looked like those shiny caps worn by film actors in the ancient 1950s films. "Well, I'll get you a nice fashionable one from Vidal Sassoon, shall I?"

He laughed out loud and I was amazed as always at how soon he cheered up. An hour later, wearing a jaunty new hat which reminded me of how handsome his father had looked on our first date on a winter's night in Sheffield in 1952, and clutching four reciprocal bunches of daffodils I'd bought for him from a Leather Lane flower seller around the corner, he set off by taxi to Waterloo Station to visit his four dancing girls from Fleet.

Meanwhile, I took the tube to Euston Station to meet Peter, who was coming down from Manchester for the weekend.

- 0 -

When Andrew returned home in the early evening he looked tired and despondent.

"What's up, *Boetie*?" Peter said as we cleared the dining room table and stacked the dish washer. "Didn't you enjoy your day out?"

Andrew flopped into the chair in front of the TV set.

"It was great," he said, not even looking at his brother, his voice dull

115

and flat.

Peter laughed. "I should think so too. What with all those pretty girls around you. I wish I was eighteen again."

Peter had hoped to snap Andrew out of his lethargy but it was clear that this was not going to be easy. He changed his tone. "You're not worried about Tuesday, are you?"

I too had guessed that Andrew had begun to count the hours before the start of the next chemo treatment, and I was thankful that Peter was around to help him build up the moral strength he needed to go back into Greenhow Ward.

Peter positioned himself on the edge of Andrew's chair and put his arm around his brother's shoulder. "Just look at it this way, *Boet*. Sooner you get this treatment over, sooner you'll be back on the hockey pitch."

"Yeah," Andrew said, at last breaking into a smile. "You're right, *Boetie*."

Chapter Eleven

April – May 1984

"I like bed number one the best," Andrew said, with a mischievous twinkle in his eye which had not been there a few minutes ago when we walked in through the entrance to The Middlesex. "It's got everything. Next to the window. Against the wall. And I can see the nurses all the time!"

Quickly he unpacked his bits and pieces. No TV this time, but a pile of A-level set-books, small change for the phone, and paper for writing letters. While he settled down to wait for Dr Annabel's arrival, I sat admiring the quiet efficient running of this ward.

Jo had said after her first visit that she liked what she saw, and from a top-notch ex-Sister that was praise indeed. The nurses were always alert; two or three always cruising around, always anticipating the patients' needs. There was an aura of special watchfulness, a warmth, a friendliness, an empathy that set them apart from others I had seen.

I wondered if this was because of the particular poignancy in people's minds about a cancer patient, which always stirs the emotions. Or was it due solely to the singular personality of the little green-eyed Sister who undoubtedly influenced the nurses working with her?

I will never forget the first time I saw her kneeling at Andrew's bedside. She was holding his hand and talking to him with her head close to his. Andrew said it made him feel she really cared, and that he was not alone.

After the first shock of confronting Dr Annabel following his gory dream of her sawing off his leg, Andrew astounded both himself and the young doctor by behaving like a model patient. Blood test, no problem. Drip, up first time.

I was impressed by his change in attitude.

"Mum," he said, with that hauntingly wistful look he had recently acquired and which made him look far older than he was. "I was

117

ashamed of the fuss I made last time. It's terribly embarrassing. I don't want to cause all that trouble again. So this time I kept telling myself over and over again it was up to me to make it work."

He had done a fantastic job of 'language behaviour', my father's behavioural science term for talking oneself into doing something, using actual out-loud speech rather than mere thoughts. The trick is that for some psychological reason once you hear your own voice commanding you out loud to do something, the response is such that you cannot let yourself down, and the task is accomplished. Mere thoughts, on the other hand, can all too easily vanish in a puff of air. This method had enabled Andrew to face an ordeal far more terrifying than even I could recognise at the time.

Dr Annabel got the pre-med just right. On went the dreaded ice-cap, in went the chemo injection. A team effort. A triumph. Andrew still hated it but he tolerated the whole session far better than before.

An observant Dr Jelliffe demonstrated his skill and knowledge of human behaviour when he spotted the ideal moment during this period to tell Andrew he might lose his leg after all, but only at the end of the week did Andrew casually mention this to me.

"Mum, I was speechless when he told me. I wonder why they didn't tell me right at the beginning." He breathed in deeply, then let the air out slowly as he held my gaze. "But you know what, I don't believe for one minute it'll happen."

All credit to Dr Jelliffe.

But sometimes, when the doubt crept back into his mind, Annabel would loosen her hair and wield her nightmare saw, and Andrew would wake up screaming.

I was not surprised to see a bond developing between him and the young Dr Annabel; an affinity born out of their common goal, each one wishing to please the other and show that they were trying hard.

If only it could have lasted. If only she could have stayed on the ward. If only he could have had one special, easily accessible doctor throughout his illness. Someone he could always go to for the continued friendship that was needed for total cooperation from a patient who was not only threatened with a fatal illness, but faced with drastic surgery and treatment by drugs that had the potential to kill.

I was angry that there was no such doctor, for it put an added responsibility on me when often I would be at a loss to know how to react and what to do next in a crisis.

118

Each morning I sat with Andrew, sometimes on his bed, sometimes next to it. Sometimes I held his hand. Sometimes I jotted down notes. If he woke up I gave him a sip of water and he would quickly go back to sleep. In the afternoons I came back in time for the pre-med, and I was always there for the chemo injection.

"Don't go, Mum,' he would murmur in his sleep if he suspected I was restless. In Greenhow there was, thank goodness, no restriction on visiting hours.

- 0 -

It is a strange anomaly of life that tragedy does not leave only sadness in its wake. It is as though nature feels she has a debt to pay after dealing a cruel blow. In spite of his own predicament, imperceptibly Andrew was changing: nature had already started bestowing on him a gift of compassion, a greater concern for other people's plights than his own which in his more lucid moments he would constantly display. It seemed that his own desperate need for help had begun to stir in him an awareness of other people's need for help. Because he was suffering he became disturbed that others suffered too.

My own compensation was a gift of acute awareness: of the world we live in, of people, of love, of beauty; of the fragility of life and the necessity not to take any of it for granted but to savour all its delights because you never knew when they would end. How incredible that the intense emotions of anguish and sorrow were actually heightening the beauty of everything I encountered, making me feel ecstasy when I went to the ballet, joy close to pain when I listened to fine music. How incredible that I was able to experience such feelings alongside my feelings of anger and despair and guilt.

It was as though I had previously been walking in a mist, taking everything for granted, feeling neither extreme sorrow nor extreme joy. Now, so many things were being revealed to me that might for ever have remained hidden.

It was years since I'd been in England in April. Hobbling past the trees and shrubs lining my route to the hospital, I felt I was part of a unique pageant in which nature's artist was daily dipping her brush into a delicate palette of pale green and yellow, creating a fantasy of feathery foliage; creating in tantalising slow motion the birth of spring.

- 0 -

On Friday Laura arrived at four o'clock. The afternoon sun shafting through the window ignited her auburn hair, and with her eyes sparkling and her cheeks glowing with excitement, I had never seen her look so lovely.

She greeted me warmly. Her smile was infectious and I wondered why it was that I'd ever had slight reservations about her attitude towards me, or could possibly have felt jealous about her involvement with Andrew.

"I've taken a week's leave," she whispered, out of Andrew's hearing. "I'm hoping to dissuade Andrew from going back to school. I can help you look after him. He'll be much better off at home."

Such love. Such genuine concern. I smiled back at her and nodded, but said nothing. She had been to see him every day, sometimes twice a day if only for a few minutes, sitting close to him, holding his hand and murmuring heaven knows what sweet nothings in his ear. But like all his other visitors she seldom got much response because most of the time he didn't even hear her.

I watched her futile attempts at persuasion and felt a pang in my heart for what she must be feeling. Sadly I wondered if in spite of their love for each other it was not the right time nor the right place for them. Perhaps their love was doomed never to come to fruition, even though Andrew was so hungry for love.

Groggily he tried to get out of bed, impatient to get home to prepare for the planned twelve days at school.

"Get back into bed, Andrew!" Sister ordered firmly, all four foot eleven of her trim little body proclaiming her authority as she marched towards his bed. "You're in no fit state to go home now. Maybe tomorrow."

Saturday and Sunday were lost days for Andrew. He was still nauseous and developed a sudden acute pain in his leg. Laura lost her battle and on Monday he forced himself out of bed in order to go to Bradfield College.

"I wish you weren't going," I said as we waited for the car I'd arranged to take him to school.

120

He rinsed his mouth after another bout of vomiting. "Stop fussing, Mum. It's nothing. Just a slight pain. I'm going and that's that. These twelve days will be the last I'll ever spend at Bradfield. I can't possibly miss them. It's too important."

"More important than seeing Laura?" I asked quietly, tentatively, having noticed what appeared to me a recent slight cooling down on his part.

"This is the final term, Mum. I may never see Simon and Stuart and James again. Please. Don't stop me."

Yes, I thought sadly. The end of his childhood. The end of being a school-boy.

The end of an era.

Angrily I reflected that he was being cheated out of ending that era with the A-level qualifications his years of first class schooling had prepared him for. Cheated out of the qualifications which would equip him to realise his goals and aspirations in life. Cheated of the chance to proceed normally along the path he had mapped for himself towards a career as a flying officer in the RAF, a career that was first kindled by his father's love of flying, which at age eight became a burning desire – "I'm going to be a pilot when I grow up" – and was then fanned into certainty at the tender age of nine by listening to a friend of ours who was a member of the illustrious 'Dam Busters' team.

He was also being cheated out of the enjoyment of his final year, and of being with the friends he held so dearly.

I glanced at him and my heart contracted, as it so often did these days. He looked so pitiful and so vulnerable and I was fearful of the reactions of the boys at school.

"I wish you'd agreed to have the Vidal Sassoon wig," I said, aware of the thoughtless cruelty of which boys are capable. "Won't you feel self-conscious when the boys look at you?"

As he laughed, his sunken eyes creased at the corners, like those of an old man.

"They'll be surprised when they first see a bald Andrew but they'll soon get used to it. If they don't, I won't mind. This is me." He shrugged and pointed to the few remaining straw-like wisps that still clung to his scalp. "It wouldn't be me in a wig!" And he laughed again with a resigned cynicism which belied his meagre eighteen years.

The car took us deep into the awakening spring countryside. Berkshire was at its most beautiful, the school like a fairy-tale castle in a shimmering sylvan setting of woods and forests and fields of emerald green.

Hillside House, adjacent to Bradfield's incredibly authentic looking open-air Greek theatre, is an old red-brick building next to one of the many acres of school playing fields. When we arrived all was quiet. We pushed open the heavy wooden door and no sooner had we stepped onto the black and red quarry tiled floor than crowds of boys came pouring down the old oak staircase and from the ground floor studies to welcome Andrew.

The special big room on the ground floor which the housemaster's wife had prepared for him was soon full of his friends. I smothered a tear of relief to see how effortlessly he made them all feel at ease, laughing at himself and his bald head and his thin useless leg, demonstrating how fast he could walk with his crutches – an amazing social skill for one so young – and how readily the boys responded in making him feel that he was no different.

That he still belonged.

- 0 -

During those twelve days we spoke on the phone every day.

"You've no idea how great it is to be back here, Mum. Everyone is being so supportive." The enjoyment helped to make him feel better far more quickly than before. He even found time for his weekly letter home to his father in Zambia:

But he did defy the doctor's orders.

Dear Dad,

I hope all is going well for you all on your tod in Lusaka. It's certainly got to be better than the way my life is going. Not that I'm having any hassle or anything. It's just that it's rather a pain being here at school with doctor's orders not to do the things I would really like to do, like some proper swimming training or a game of tennis when I get a spare moment in the afternoons.

It was great to speak to you on the phone last night. I can't remember whether I told you I was having some pain in my leg. Well, anyway, Mum phoned Dr Jelliffe today and asked him about this. Apparently it's quite normal. The pain is being caused by the collection of dead cells after the chemo has taken effect. I have some swelling below the knee as well, but I'm going to have another scan after the next shots of chemo, just to check up on how things are going.

I attended my A-level classes today and found it exhausting enough getting there, let alone trying to concentrate on the work. I've missed so much, it's unbelievable.

Having looked at the dates of my English exams, I've decided to ask my housemaster about the possibility of writing them in hospital, as I'll still be stuck in bed then. What do you think?

Do you know yet when you'll be able to come over here again? I do hope it's soon! I miss you so much.

Tons of love,

Andrew XXX

He took part in a swimming match against another school!

Fortunately no harm was done, though I shuddered to think of the danger of fracturing the tibia which was becoming very brittle as the tumour shrank, leaving in its wake that mass of dead cells.

That wasn't all. Later I learned from the mother of a boy several years junior to Andrew, that during those twelve days Andrew had devoted all his spare time to coaching younger boys. He had taught her son to do the butterfly stroke, and all the boys had regarded him as their hero.

They needed help and he was helping them.

Another highlight was being invited by the shooting team to take up his former place in the School Eight, this time for a full-bore rifle meeting at Bisley. Bursting with pride I watched him boost his team's success, thankful that you don't need two legs to shoot a target.

123

A happy time, but for Andrew the best part of that brief idyll was being able to talk about his plight with Stuart, Simon and James. Far more important than talking to me about it. Or even to Laura.

"I was so sad when I had to leave, Mum."

- 0 -

During those twelve days I saw all the ballet that was on in London, discovered the delights of the nearby Barbican Centre and generally feasted on the arts, something I couldn't do in the middle of Africa. I also explored the City of London, discovering an unknown richness of history on my doorstep. And a few minutes' walk from the flat was Leather Lane's colourful street market, its fascinating hustle and bustle drawing me daily to stalls filled with every imaginable item from ball gowns to boomerangs.

I walked for miles but every step I took was still painful.

And because of this I had a momentous encounter which opened up an exciting new perception for me.

One morning I was having a quick cup of tea with Jo Rodin.

"There's a friend of mine I want you to see", she said, fixing me with her direct gaze. "She's an ex-nurse who is now doing reflex therapy of the feet. She's very much into alternative medicine. I'm sure she'll be able to help."

That very afternoon I phoned for an appointment. Next day I took the tube to Euston Square. The reflexology lady had soft brown hair and a soft lilting voice. Her hands when she spread the oil on my feet were soft and soothing beyond belief, but the moment she began massaging my feet I knew this was no ordinary, soft person.

She spoke to me about Andrew, Jo having told her all about him, and I suspect that Jo may have sent me to her for this reason rather than for my ailing feet.

One exciting concept captured my imagination.

"It's the patient who decides to sing his own song who gets better from cancer," she said. "The patient who takes a positive role in his own treatment."

I thought about this long and hard. It made a great deal of sense to me. On her recommendation I attended some exhilarating meetings and lectures which enforced what my father had instilled in me: that the mind cannot be separated from the body and no disease is ever

124

entirely physical.

The lessons I was learning were electrifying. I became totally convinced that if Andrew could rediscover a zest for life, an enjoyment of life, and a brand new meaning to his life, he would have the incentive to reassemble the shattered pieces and *sing his own song*.

In the beginning, the foot therapy lady told me, I would have to help him to do this by always presenting a positive stance. It was necessary for him to know that I cared enough and believed without any doubt whatsoever that he would survive. It would be this knowing that would have a positive impact on his own determination to fight. I would be the catalyst for his own actions, the foot therapy lady said, but he would be the one who would replace despair with a positive and optimistic outlook, with control of his own body, generating the power to command it to reject and destroy the tumour.

Command your body to reject and destroy the tumour?

Could this really happen?

I said it out loud to myself and it sounded like a bit of a crackpot idea. Did the body really have that kind of power?

Well, we would have to find out.

And after all, wasn't it very similar in concept to my father's theory of 'language behaviour'? Where you tell yourself out loud to do something or not to do something, and there is no way you can then let yourself down, so you carry out the instruction to the letter?

The foot reflexology lady had opened a door that gave an extra dimension to the new goal in my life.

The goal to save Andrew's life.

- 0 -

Andrew phoned every day to tell me of the day's events at school and to make sure that I was all right.

He was worried about *me!*

This concern for my well-being was part of the new awareness he was developing that was manifesting in his thoughtfulness for other people.

Again I caught in his voice the intense enjoyment he was experiencing at being at school. He was savouring every moment of his twelve precious days. Yet, though he never once mentioned going back into hospital on Tuesday, I knew just how afraid he was at the prospect

125

of the third chemotherapy treatment.

Chapter Twelve

May 1984
(from Andrew's diary)

Approaching The Middlesex, the nausea sets in.
I know what'll happen which makes it all worse.
I say out loud I feel better but it never works.
I don't want to do this any more.

The lift to the ward takes forever.
The doors clunk back. We step out.
Mum is beside me, carrying my bag
Slowly we walk through the doors.

My bed is prepared
The drip stand is ready.
The nurses greet me like a friend.
They know what will happen and yet are so calm!

Into pyjamas
and the horror begins.
Questions are asked, and then it's the needles.
The blood tests first

The doctor arrives.
How are you, Andrew?
I want to say awful, I don't want to be here
But I smile and say thank you, I'm fine.

The cannula inserted
The saline infused.
My bladder fills. I hold on as long as I can

Until I must take my drip with me to ease the pain.

I return
And they're there with that thing –
The ice-cap, cold, hard, and heartless,
I hate it. It smirks, ready to inflict its torture.

On it goes. I vomit, I know what comes next.
The nurses are angels
They try hard to calm me
The doctor is called. We'll sedate you, Andrew, so it
   won't be so bad.

They try
Again and again
But always I must struggle
To be in control.

The doctor arrives. In her hand a syringe
Larger than life.
I'm not a horse, you know!
And she laughs.

Please, put it in slowly. Don't hurt me, I plead!
And in goes pink poison
that will keep me alive.
At last I drift off. Soon it will end.

They come and they go
It seems like a lifetime but it's only three days.
In goes the fluid
The drips are changed.

The ice cap comes off and goes on
More nausea and vomiting
Please God, when will it end?
The drip comes down.

You can go now, Andrew.

I'm weak. I'm alive!
But I know it's not over and soon
It will happen again ...

- 0 -

He was in a side ward this time, a starkly bare but light and airy room off the main ward, with two large windows facing a mish-mash of old Victorian buildings. Apart from the bed, a bedside table and a chair, there was a wash basin and – surprise surprise – a television set.

Five minutes later Dr Annabel appeared in the doorway.

"Hello, Andrew," she said, walking quickly to his bedside, her blonde tresses neatly compressed into a shiny bun on top of her head.

"Hi!" he said, smiling from ear to ear, so happy to see her.

"I've just popped in for a minute," she said. "I'm no longer on this ward but if there's anything I can do to help, please let me know."

Andrew's smile faded, as though someone above him had let the strings drop.

The rotation system was obviously necessary for their training but this was the first indication Andrew had that in a teaching hospital doctors are moved frequently from one department to another.

I sat watching the silent exchange flow between Andrew and Annabel. Her hands were tied but she clearly knew how much he had grown to depend on her. She must also have seen, just as I did, how sad he was to lose her.

He held his head in his hands. "I don't believe it, Mum," he said after she had gone. "How can she leave me now?"

How indeed, I thought, knowing there was nothing I could do about it either.

A few minutes later Dr Mike burst through the doorway like a whirling dervish, his white coat flying, his broad smile just for Andrew.

He did a great job in compensating for Andrew's disappointment at losing Annabel. A cuddly sort of person, softly spoken though energetic and alert, he looked about twenty-eight, a small man in height but a giant at heart. He treated Andrew as though he was a very important person, calling him 'Boss' and always seeking his approval.

And he soon won Andrew's trust.

His methods were different from Annabel's, but Andrew mercifully slept through most of the treatment, though this might have been

129

partly due to the quietness of the private room.

I asked Andrew if he liked being on his own.

He shook his head. "It was okay for a while, but I miss seeing the nurses all the time. I have to ring the bell now. In the main ward they were always there for me."

Walking through the main ward that afternoon, I noticed Tom in bed number one. He was asleep but I stood next to him for a few minutes, my hand resting lightly on his arm. He was an eighteen year old boy also suffering from osteosarcoma, but I had never seen him with any visitors. He and Andrew were neck and neck in their treatment. They compared notes, and there was a special bond of empathy between them.

Tom was docile and gentle, quiet and unassuming. He didn't ever complain.

"I don't know how he puts up with the chemo the way he does," Andrew said when I told him I'd seen Tom. "It doesn't matter what they do to him. He just lies there and takes it."

"He sets a very good example," I said pointedly, though I did wonder why this time the two boys had been separated.

As I walked through the ward towards Andrew's room the following morning I noticed that bed number one was empty.

Oh no! My heart stopped beating. I swallowed hard. "Has Tom gone home?" I asked a nurse, biting my lip.

The nurse hastened to reassure me. "Tom? He's been transferred to Dressmakers Ward for surgery tomorrow."

She walked with me to Andrew's door. "He's waiting for you. He's just about to have his pre-med."

Like a recurring nightmare it all happened. The ice-cap. The injection. The brown paper bag. I prayed he would stay asleep.

"I'm glad you're here, Mum," I heard him whisper.

My nearness soothed him through the nausea. At the end of the long day I tiptoed out.

As I unlocked my front door I heard the phone ring.

"Andrew is awake," the night nurse said. "He's feeling very low. Please, could you come back right away?"

"Middlesex Hospital," I said to the taxi, then bit into the apple I had grabbed for my supper.

His door was wide open. I crept in.

He opened his eyes, reached for my hand, sighed then closed them again.

I stayed with him for over an hour, repeating softly all the positive thoughts that came into my head, feeling the tension drain from his body as it drained from mine. Then gently I withdrew my hand and tiptoed out again.

I took a taxi home, my thoughts still with Andrew. Everyone is doing their utmost to keep his morale high. Get-well cards arrive every day and visitors are many. Laura pops in whenever she can and I pop out to window-shop in order to leave them alone. Dr Mike is very supportive. He treats Andrew with great respect. Never talks down at him and never reprimands him. He is a very good doctor. Andrew says they are chums. Why then, with so many things going our way, does such a pall of gloom hang over us now? Why is there this great big black cloud without a single break through which the sun can shine?

- 0 -

The dream filled my night with terror and I woke in the morning fraught with guilt. But there was no time to waste. I had to get to the hospital quickly.

I jumped off the bus in Oxford Street, right opposite Berners Street, the road leading directly up to The Middlesex. For a moment I stood looking northwards towards the Post Office Tower soaring into the sky behind the hospital. The hospital was straight ahead of me, at the far end of Berners Street, majestic and imposing, like a temple at the end of a tunnel. The source of our darkness. And of our light. The place that had become our second home.

I took a deep breath and started walking.

Each day the distance seemed longer. I hobbled on, slower and slower but I had to be there for Andrew.

In Greenhow Ward there was much hilarity. The little green-eyed Sister was cutting a cake.

"What's the occasion?" I asked, accepting a tiny piece.

"Dr Mike got married this morning! He's in there now, with Andrew."

Most people take at least a day off to get married, but not Mike. Here he was, getting things ready and talking all the time in soft tones to Andrew. Dedicated.

I put the flask of orange juice on the bedside table. Andrew hardly

131

ate anything while he was having chemo, so I brought in things I knew he liked, as well as the juice I squeezed from the oranges I bought every day in Leather Lane. Not only delicious, but full of vitamin C.

I sat down and forced myself into a trance-like state.

- 0 -

The ritual begins.

Ice-cap ... needle ... brown paper bag ...

Nausea ...

Invisible and silent I watch.

Andrew knows I am here.

- 0 -

At last he was quiet. As he slept I noticed how thin he was.

Can he survive with so little body weight, I wondered.

His eyes, circled by charcoal rings, lay deep in his face, the few remaining hairs on his head, dry and white, adding to the old, wizened look. Laura had tried to persuade him to have the wisps cut short, but he was adamant they should remain as they were.

At seven I went home.

- 0 -

I arrive next morning earlier than usual and decide to visit Tom in Dressmakers Ward. His replacement knee and tibia operation is the same as the one Andrew will have on the seventh of June, so it will be interesting to see how he is coping on his first post-operative day. I have never seen anyone else visit Tom, so I am sure I will not be in the way.

I buy a box of chocolates at the hospital shop and go up in the clanking lift to Dressmakers. Tom is in the fourth bed down, on the right hand side.

There is a huge cage over his leg. His eyes are closed and I rest my hand gently on his shoulder, in case he is awake.

"Tom," I whisper.

He opens his eyes. He says nothing and I wonder if in the aftermath of the anaesthetic he is able to recognise me.

132

"Tom, it's Andrew's mum. How are you? I've brought you some chocolates."

He smiles.

Not a full smile. More with his eyes than with his mouth.

He looks at the chocolates and nods, smiles again but still does not say a word.

I pull up a stool next to him. His big dark eyes look up at me. He has the same gentle look in them that he always has but now they are sad too.

"I have a lot of pain in my foot," he says at last.

I think how brave he is. How alone.

He takes my hand.

Places it under the cage.

On the empty space ...

... where once his leg had been.

- 0 -

I sat by Andrew's bed, keeping a close watch on his face and on the drip. When I saw it becoming irregular, or stopping, I rang the bell. It was a small contribution but it made me feel useful.

Suddenly the arm and hand began to swell, as though it was being pumped up by a bicycle pump. I was still stunned by what had happened to Tom and terrified that something dreadful would also happen to Andrew.

The nurses rushed in. They called Sister. They bleeped Mike and in a flash he appeared.

I flattened myself against the wall.

The arm and hand were swelling by the minute.

Mike took one look.

"Quick! Take down the drip!"

The nurses flew into action then all stood round the bed and watched.

No one moved until the swelling began to subside.

Mike saw my look of fear, my incomprehension.

"Instead of the fluid going into the vein it was starting to break through the walls of the vein into the surrounding tissues," he explained. "This 'tissueing' can be extremely dangerous. It can do irreparable damage if allowed to continue."

133

I gulped. No wonder there was panic. "Will you start again when the arm is back to normal?" I asked.

He shook his head. "I'm afraid not. So to compensate for the lack of fluids to his body, essential as you know for its recovery from the chemo drugs and to ensure no permanent damage to his kidneys, Andrew must now take a great deal of water by mouth." He raised his eyebrows, then smiled. "If you like, we can leave you here to be in charge of that."

Not as easy as it sounded because Andrew was semi-comatose. Tears welled in my eyes. Would I be able to do this properly? And yet I had a glowing feeling that Mike should have such faith in me.

Every half-hour I filled the glass and held it to his lips. Supporting his head was difficult. When the water ran down his chin and soaked his pyjamas I was frantic. I was terrified of not giving him enough. But it was also strangely satisfying to be doing something positive for a change, instead of always playing a passive role at the hospital.

I sat staring at his face. An eerie stillness crept in around me. The night noises were distant and muffled as they echoed down the empty passages.

Not daring to look away for one moment, I was suddenly conscious for the first time in many years of him once having been a part of me. I remembered the joy of bringing him home from the hospital. Of holding him on my knee, supporting his wobbling head, and Adam, our Zambian cook, his eyes wide with wonder, kneeling down in front of the tiny baby. "He is beautiful," he had whispered, and I had looked at my son's blue eyes and the perfect, round head with its silver blond sheen, and I had smiled a smile of total happiness and pride.

Eventually the nurses took over. They said I looked exhausted and told me to go home.

Yes, I was exhausted, but like so many other nights, the moment my head hit the pillow my fears and my guilt flooded the screen of my mind. Reluctantly I took one of the sleeping tablets Philip had given me; without it I could not have kept going.

- 0 -

Andrew had to stay in hospital until Sunday to make sure he was sufficiently hydrated, but he was determined to go to school on Monday as planned. He was very weak, very thin, very pale and very

134

sick, but he did not care. School was drawing him back like a magnet. Right now he thought this second visit would definitely be his last and nothing was going to stop him.

Maybe our nomadic life was to blame for this need. We had moved house so many times, but no matter which house or town we lived in, 'school' was always there, in the same place with the same people, forming a solid base in which he felt secure. Soon this solid base would no longer be his haven; he would be an 'old boy'. So for him it was vital not to miss one single precious day. He was not to know then that something dramatic and unexpected would make it possible for him to return yet again in July for the final few days of the term.

- 0 -

During these brief visits the housemaster and his wife lavished extra attention on Andrew, saw that he ate well and was comfortable and warm, and provided him with moral support. So did Simon, Stuart and James, and in the midst of his terrible ordeal it was a happy time for Andrew.

- 0 -

Once again left on my own, the dream returned to haunt me and often I was afraid to go to bed. Then suddenly I had a brainwave.

Ahead of me were almost two free weeks. What about trying to take my O-level Spanish examination, which I had cancelled when Andrew became ill?

Next day I went to the University of London Examination Department in Russell Square, where a kind man bent the rules to fit me in.

I bought a set of Spanish tapes and carried the recorder wherever I went. I fell asleep listening to it. Woke up to it. Switched it on in the buses and on the tubes and had imaginary Spanish conversations with passers-by while walking down the streets.

It stopped me thinking about Andrew all the time, wondering whether he would have the same fate as Tom, and mercifully the dream receded.

I soon regained my former linguistic competence and was sure I would get an 'A'.

There was only one problem.

In a blank moment I had not connected the date of the first paper with the day Andrew would be admitted to The Middlesex for his crucial leg-saving operation.

Chapter Thirteen

June 1984

Writing a Spanish examination when my husband was arriving at Heathrow Airport and my son was being admitted to hospital for surgery that could result in losing a leg, was probably the craziest thing I ever did in my life. And like the dream I once had in which I walked on to the platform of the Cape Town City Hall and sat down in front of a gaping Steinway piano, hoping it would swallow me up before I had to play Beethoven's 3rd piano concerto with a full orchestra, when the only thing I knew was a one-finger version of Charlie Chaplin's hauntingly beautiful theme music for Limelight, there was no way I could succeed.

I looked around at the sea of bent heads. Pens scribbling confidently. Pages flicking over.

What on earth was I doing here?

As my irrational feelings of inadequacy as a mother screamed at me, so they obliterated every Spanish verb from my mind; but I stuck it out. At the end of two hours I careered down the steps and ran like an escaped convict all the way to The Middlesex.

"Hi, Mum, how did you do?" Andrew said as I staggered purple-faced into Dressmakers Ward. He was already tucked up neatly in bed. Colin had picked him up from school in the company car that had collected him from the airport.

"Like an idiot," I said, flopping into Colin's arms.

It was wonderful to be close to Colin, but I couldn't help it – my eyes strayed first to Andrew. How frail he looked! How vulnerable. How angular the contours of his face. How grey his skin against the white of the sheets.

I was filled with fear.

Andrew was frightened too, not that he said anything to betray this. But I knew by his increasing bad temper and his uncommunicative attitude that he was.

137

A busy schedule lay ahead.

First on the list was the NMR scan at the Hammersmith. That night at supper Colin poured us each a glass of wine.

"It was unbelievable," he said, smiling from ear to ear. "The tumour has actually shrunk. I saw it with my own eyes. It's much smaller than it was in March."

I breathed out deeply, savouring the sound of the words which were like music to my ears.

Shrunk. Smaller. Shrunk. Smaller. Shrunk ...

I raised my glass. "This means they can go ahead on Thursday, doesn't it? Knowing that because the tumour hasn't got any larger, it probably hasn't spread to those vital tendons?"

I took a large gulp of my wine. "Come on, Col. This will surely push him into Dr Jelliffe's eighty-five percent safe haven. Won't it, darling?"

Colin was suddenly too choked up to reply. For a few moments we sat in silence. Then in a quiet voice he reminded me of Dr Jelliffe's warning.

"*Even the scan can't give us the vital information we need about the state of the tendons, the arteries and the muscles,*" he quoted in a hushed monotone.

I lay in bed that night, trying hard to think positively but in spite of the good news the dream came back to haunt me in all its lurid Technicolor horror.

- 0 -

Back at The Middlesex all other tests and X-rays were completed. Everything appeared to be in order and the operation would proceed as planned: On Thursday. At eight in the morning. The first on the list.

But there was one other routine formality to be completed.

The consent form.

He was eighteen. Officially an adult.

He would have to sign it himself.

When Dr Jelliffe had told him in April that the leg might have to be amputated, he had accepted it like a man. No, he had *faced* it like a man. Lately he had rarely mentioned it, yet whenever I heard his muffled screams at night and rushed into his room to calm him down, it was always the same nightmare.

Annabel sawing off his leg.

Now, suddenly, the bare facts were staring him in the face.

- 0 -

It was the evening visiting hour. The night before the op. When we walked in at seven sharp we found him in an ugly and depressed mood.

Colin sat down next to him and put his arm around his shoulders.

"What's wrong, son?

Andrew slowly shook his head. "The houseman came to see me. He had this ... this piece of paper in his hand. He asked me to sign it."

"What did it say?"

He took a deep breath. His words came jerkily, as though from an automated recording.

"I agree. To the amputation. Of my leg. If. While undergoing the operation. This is found. To be necessary."

I closed my eyes and opened them again quickly. "Did you sign it?"

"It was so sudden, Mum. I panicked. I didn't know what to do. It was the most difficult decision I've ever had to make. I almost didn't sign it."

I was numb with the horror of Andrew's fear, as though it were my own. I knew that even though the virtues of the modern artificial leg had been explained to him, giving permission to cut off his leg had taken more guts than I could ever have imagined having.

I knew something else too.

In signing that form Andrew had become a man.

A real man.

- 0 -

I couldn't sleep.
I sat up in bed.
It was dark. The other patients sleeping
Some were snoring.

I threw off the bedclothes,

139

Stared at my leg. I rubbed my foot.
Would it still be there tomorrow?

In the morning I talked to the nurses
Waylaid them one by one as they passed my bed.
I didn't want to be alone.

- 0 -

We had intended going to the hospital early on Thursday morning to monitor the progress of the operation. The Graysons had told us that Paul's operation a year and a half ago had taken five hours, so it would be a long wait.

But our guardian angel – Jo Rodin – put her foot down.

"It won't do any good to hang around the hospital. You'll only be in the way. There'll be nothing you can do."

The oracle had spoken.

- 0 -

The front door bell rings. Still half dead after one of Philip's sleeping tablets I stagger to the door.

It is Jo. And unexpectedly also on the doorstep, our old ex-RAF friend Hans Haslett, retired chief pilot from our Williamson Diamonds days in Tanzania. He has known Andrew since he was a baby and is very fond of him. He knows how badly Andrew wanted to be a pilot in the RAF.

I make a pot of tea. We drink several cups each, then take turns making fresh ones, even though it is coming out of our ears.

Jo sits next to the phone and answers all the calls. She tells them we are busy. She is polite to everyone but cuts them short, telling them the line must be kept open.

We talk about the hot weather, the Labour Party and the Conservatives, the new Italian restaurant in Farringdon Road around the corner – anything to keep our minds off what the surgeons might have to do.

The suspense is unbearable. Worse than anything I have ever known.

I close my eyes. I drift. I am sitting on the edge of a cliff, looking

140

down. Waves crash on rocks below. A big black void sucks me down but just as I am about to reach the bottom I float up again and suddenly I am in the Operating Theatre. There are bright lights and there is a strange noise coming from the operating table.

Mr Sweetnam is there. And Dr Jelliffe. Dr Annabel too. At least I think it is them but it's hard to be sure with those strange green suits they are wearing, and those green masks with only their eyes peeping through like some strange creatures from Mars.

I breathe in short sharp gasps. Will the tumour be too close to the vital blood vessels and the tendons and the muscles needed for the leg to survive, I wonder. And if they are, what will the men in green do first?

They all have scalpels in their hands. Some are fine and straight. Some are thick and curved – like my hunting knife.

One is a saw.

Mr Sweetnam's weapon is the first one to move. His scalpel starts at the top of the leg and scores a clean straight line down to the ankle. The flesh parts. Blood spurts everywhere, spraying into the wind and mixing with the rain that is falling down in sheets, down the edge of the cliff.

Dr Jelliffe is next. He lifts his scalpel which is small and thin and straight. He deftly makes a cut then stands back, his green suit drenched with blood.

Annabel steps forward. She lifts her saw and I pray, the way I have lately learned to pray, to anyone who will listen. I remind myself that Andrew's bedside table and the walls next to his bed are covered with get-well cards stuck on with Blue Tack. He has the good wishes of everyone we know and some we don't know. Surely with such concentrated concern from so many people, Annabel will stop ...

He even has a letter from a friend in Zambia, a devoutly religious woman who had called a special meeting of her church group in order to pray for him. She had passed her letter round the entire group before posting it to Andrew. Each one had laid their healing hands on it and she told Andrew if he held the letter against his leg he would receive the healing powers. Once or twice I discovered this precious letter under his sheet, way down at the bottom of the bed, crumpled to the shape of his leg.

One by one the minutes tick by. They stretch the morning into an eternity. Even Jo, who is trained not to show her emotion or her anxiety, is clearly agitated.

She looks at her watch.

"It's one o'clock," she says.

Five hours have passed.

She picks up the phone. I watch her dial the number. Oh how well I know it.

Colin and I hold hands. We dare not look at one another. Hans stares at the wall.

Time stands still.

Jo asks to be put through to the recovery room in the theatre ...

"Could you please tell me if Andrew is out of theatre?" she says.

Nobody breathes.

Still holding the phone Jo glares at the wall, her eyes wide as saucers as she waits.

Then she mouths to us: "He is out of theatre!"

"And could you please tell me if the prosthesis was inserted in his leg?"

The blood drains from my head. I am sitting on the edge of that cliff and all I can see is Tom with his big sad dark eyes and the empty space in the cage.

Suddenly Jo's hand shoots up and her thumb shoots up after it and her face breaks into a huge grin and I am falling off the cliff ...

My limbs drift away. My insides explode.

Jo puts down the phone and at last she looks at us. It is a long slow look with a smile that spreads gradually from her eyes, down and over her cheeks to her cherry shaped mouth. Then suddenly everything snaps into focus and we all leap to our feet, jumping and shouting and yelling with joy and relief. We hug each other over and over again, hurling ourselves at each other like football players who have just scored a goal.

Jo takes a deep breath. "I must phone Philip", she says, and her eyes light up as she tells him the wonderful news.

I imagine Philip's face: At first it has a peaceful, serene look, a look of calm and fulfilment, a look of love and human understanding. As he listens a slow quiet smile spreads outwards and upwards. His eyes are like stars that transform his face into a galaxy of joy.

- 0 -

After we had made a few phone calls ourselves, and simmered down a bit, Colin poured the celebratory drinks. A hefty Croft Original on the rocks for Jo and me, and a beer for himself and Hans.

Jo saw me looking at my watch. "You can't see Andrew yet," she said softly. "He'll still be in the recovery room."

We bowed to her superior knowledge, but how we managed to contain ourselves until the evening visiting session at seven o'clock, I do not know.

- 0 -

Andrew is still out cold. We sit at the sides of his bed. Watching. His thin face is as white as the sheet. His mouth parched and puckered. His cheeks sunken.

There is an enormous cage over his leg, exactly like the one Tom had. Tubes and drips and draining bags are everywhere. I shudder. Fleetingly I see Annabel and her saw, then I take a deep breath and slowly breathe out.

Colin whispers: "I don't suppose Jo could have got it wrong, could she?"

How is it that I am thinking exactly the same thing? I'd even been on the point of saying it. They say that if two people live together for long enough their minds work in unison. Or are we in some way psychic?

I shake my head, still thinking about Tom. If anyone besides me had visited Tom after his operation, did they wonder too? Did anyone sit at his bedside and weep? What would we be thinking now if Mr Sweetnam had not been able to reconstruct the leg, skilfully and miraculously and unbelievably brilliantly, sawing away the diseased bone (was that the strange noise I heard on the cliff?) and inserting the metal prosthesis and tying up the myriad blood vessels and muscles that make up the human leg? What would we be doing now?

We sit silently. For half an hour we gaze at him. He does not move. Not even an eyelid flickers. Nearly every patient in the ward has had an operation today, and occasionally we smile and nod at the other silent visitors.

Colin is on one side of the bed. I am on the other. Almost as though we had rehearsed it our hands move towards the cage. He catches my eye. I smile. Then knowing what we are going to do, even knowing

143

before we touch the cover, we lift it and look.

And there it is!

Enormously encased in mounds of dressings and bandages.

Straight and still and whole and solid.

It is Andrew's leg.

Before we leave, Colin takes one of his business cards from his pocket. He slides the cap off his pen. I watch his face. His eyes glisten. His lip quivers.

On the back of the card he writes a little note to Andrew.

He pins it to the pillow. It says:

I have counted your toes. And there are ten.

Love, Dad.

Chapter Fourteen

Andrew, it's all over ...
All over ...
All over ...
We'll take you back to the ward now ...
Ward now ...
Ward now ...

Andrew! Andrew, your Dad's been in
And your Mum. But you were fast asleep.
More cards for you. Flowers. I'll put them in water.

What? Dad?
When? Why didn't you wake me?

He's left something for you. A note.

A note?
Oh God, the pain. Someone do something about the
  pain. I need the toilet. Need it now! My leg?
Please, let it be there. It must be there.
No-one said it would be like this.
If it's so painful it must be there. But it might not.
Tom?
Tell me, someone.
Have I still got my leg?
I need to know
Now ...

Andrew, your Dad's left you a note
It's next to your pillow. There it is.

I reach for it, knock over my glass of water. I'm so thirsty

145

Thirsty …
Thirsty …

Strange shapes float, fade past my eyes.
Tom. I see Tom.
He walks towards me, crutches squeaking on the floor
No leg
His face getting bigger and bigger,
Grinning.
Tom!
Stop!
Don't go! Talk to me! Have I got my leg?
Tom keeps walking
Right past me, through me, though the wall,
Grinning …
Oh, poor Tom!

Andrew, here's the note. Your Dad's note.
Don't you want to read it?
I lift my head but it sinks like a stone in a swamp
Squashy. Sloshy. Squidgy.
I lift it again.
I see the card. Dad's writing. Small. Neat.
'I have counted your toes
And there are ten.
Love, Dad'

I have counted your toes and there are ten!
Oh my God! It's still there. They've done it. Dad, thank
  you. But I wish you were here now. And Mum.
Are you sure, Dad?
Are you sure?

Chapter Fifteen

We sat on the chairs in the passage outside Dressmakers Ward waiting impatiently for the stroke of three when we could go in and see Andrew again. No free visiting hours in this ward.

"I'm so excited for him," I said to Colin. "I can't wait to see his face now that he knows he still has his leg."

Colin blinked his eyes. Even though he is a tough, strong man he has a very soft soppy side to him, especially where his children are concerned. I could see that this moment was evoking in him a surge of emotion he was finding difficult to suppress.

I squeezed his hand. "I'm dying to hear what he thought when he saw the note you left on his pillow last night. He must have been over the moon with joy after all those months of worrying."

Colin squeezed my hand back, and at two minutes to three we stood up and walked to the door. My heart was thumping against my ribs. I had to make a deliberate effort to control my breathing so that I would look quite normal when I walked in. Why does one want to cry when one is happy, I asked myself, glancing at Colin and seeing that he was in the same state that I was.

At dead on three o'clock we walked into the ward to be greeted by a cantankerous Andrew.

We had expected a jubilant Andrew. We had expected him to be rejoicing in the success of the operation.

Not a bit of it. He didn't even mention Colin's little note about counting his toes, which I noticed was lying on his bedside table.

All he could think of was that he could not pass water.

Not a single drop.

Poor Andrew. He lay there with his face and shoulders twisting in agony, grasping his stomach and uttering indecipherable grumbling complaints.

I hurried out to find Sister, leaving Colin trying to cheer him up. Before I reached her office I met one of the nurses on Andrew's ward and waylaid her.

147

"It's a fairly common post-operative spasm," she explained. "We were hoping it would start again naturally but we're just about to insert a catheter." She glanced at the watch pinned upside-down to her uniform. "We'll do it as soon as visiting hour is over. Not long to go now and then he'll be far happier."

She looked at me then, and smiled. She touched my arm.

"I wish you'd seen his face when he woke up and found that note. The whole ward knew about it. We heard this shriek and we all came rushing in. He'd just woken up. I'd been in a few moments earlier to check his BP and his temperature and he'd still been fast asleep. *'Look at this!'* he yelled, holding up the note. *'I've still got my leg, I've still got my leg!'* We went along with him of course. Pretending not to know, and then I said, 'Well, let's see it then, shall we, Andrew?'."

She took a deep breath and looked up at the ceiling then carried on with her story. "I don't know when last I saw such a look on anyone's face. We all stood around. The other patients were looking on too, not saying a word, just smiling. Then very, very slowly I lifted the covers off, like in slow motion. He was holding his breath. Even I was holding my breath and I'd already seen it. As his leg appeared his eyes got wider and wider. He lay there, flopped on his pillows, kind of shaking his head and taking deep breaths and closing his eyes then opening them again as though he didn't believe what he was seeing. He read the little note from his Dad again, only this time out loud, for the whole ward to hear. Then he just said one word. *'Wow!'*."

I hugged the Sister. I couldn't help it.

"I wish I'd been here to see it," I said, feeling quite overwhelmed.

She smiled. "It cheered us all up. And the other patients too. To see someone so thrilled."

When we visited Andrew that evening he was much happier. Colin's little note was still on the bed-side table, right on the edge, within his reach. Andrew nudged his Dad and pointed at the note.

"Thank you, Dad," he said, smiling and shaking his head.

An extra plastic bag hung at the side of the bed. The relief from the catheter had been immediate he told us, and soon he became his old self.

But not for long.

Within a few days, when the initial powerful pain killers began to be tailed off, the pain in the leg became excruciating.

I was puzzled. Surely something was wrong. Why was he being

allowed to suffer such intense pain? Every person's threshold of pain is different, but wasn't the essence of good nursing to relieve that pain? Why were they not controlling it? Wasn't nursing about making people feel better?

With mounting anger I watched Andrew's face grow greyer and the dark circles under his eyes deepen. And each day my anger grew when the pain was allowed to continue even after I had spoken about it to the staff.

Then I began to realise what was happening.

Ideally, with the new pain-killing ethos, each new dose of pain-killing drugs is administered before the effect of the last one has worn off. This ensures that relief is maintained at a comfortable level. But I discovered by talking to Andrew that sometimes, if the pain killer was given in the form of an injection, he would refuse to have it.

He was in a rebellious mood, not easy for anyone to manage. As his pain persisted he became more and more perverse. Seemingly unaware of his needle phobia, and that it was this alone, and not lack of pain, that made him stoically refuse these injections, they gave him no alternative drug. This lapse allowed the pain to take over, so that the next dose was not enough to drag him out of the tortuous depths of pain into which he had sunk.

In desperation I expressed these views to one of the young doctors who was apparently also unaware of the problem. I was furious when the situation still did not improve. Why was such a blinkered approach being adopted? A similar blinkered approach was adopted by this same rule-bound young doctor when I tried in vain to get him to give Andrew Vitamin C and Vitamin E tablets to hasten the healing process.

The other problem was visiting hours. The many friends who could have kept him distracted all came at the same time and stood around the bed talking to each other rather than to Andrew. Then there were hours and hours with no visitors at all. Colin and I also had to share the precious time with all the others, and I began to lose the closeness that had earlier been established between us. On top of that, because he had to stay in bed for one whole week without getting up, Andrew could not go around the ward chatting to people as he loved to do. This might have taken his mind off the pain.

- 0 -

One afternoon when we arrived at Andrew's bedside, Mr Sweetnam was just leaving the ward. This was the first time we had seen him since the operation and we told him how delighted we were with the result.

We stood looking down at the leg which was completely encased in a huge, fat dressing. "You must not try to move it, Andrew," Mr Sweetnam said sternly, then explained that it had to be manually lifted with great care so as not to disturb the delicate reconstruction.

When he showed us the X-rays I was amazed at what they had done. There was a brief note attached to the envelope which I read out loud:

"*Resection of right upper tibial osteosarcoma. Reconstruction with a Scales endoprosthesis.* What does that mean, Mr Sweetnam?"

Mr Sweetnam spelled it out to us in layman's terms, and later I wrote it up in my notebook.

There was a metal tibia replacing three-quarters of the original tibia, with a connecting spike reaching down almost to the ankle. Above the knee, part of the femur was replaced with metal, its connecting spike reaching about a third of the way up the femur. The knee itself was replaced by a very clever hinged metal joint, pivoting on a plastic-covered rod. The top of the fibula had also been removed, since they had found in earlier cases that this tended to interfere with the new unorthodox knee joint.

But one important part remained.

The patella.

"The knee cap is the vital link for tendons and muscles," Mr Sweetnam explained, "and Andrew is fortunate that we were able to save it."

Some of the existing muscles and tendons had also been employed in the reconstruction, but not all in their conventional positions, and some muscle tissue was used to wrap around the new knee joint to give it stability. Other muscles were slightly repositioned, giving the leg its somewhat unconventional look. Plastic tendons were used where not enough had existed, and the whole knee joint was further supported by a plastic sling.

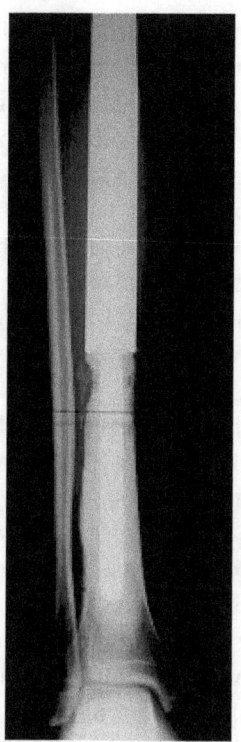

X-Ray of Mr Sweetnam's leg-saving prosthesis, June 1984

As I closed my notebook that night, I looked up at Colin.
"We are so lucky that it all went according to plan"
"It is a miracle," he answered.

- 0 -

The pain continued to dominate all other feelings Andrew might have had. The catheter was removed and his bladder returned to normal. The drips came down too, so he should now have been able to rest properly and enjoy the success of his operation.

But he did not.

I tried to rationalise that it was not surprising that there should be pain. Hadn't he had an incision almost the complete length of his leg? Three major bones severed and countless muscles, blood vessels and tendons cut, reorganised or removed and then all stitched up? This would add up to more pain than I could ever envisage.

151

In my naïve ignorance and misplaced stoicism, I endured the pain of watching his pain. I was unaware that as a mother it was my right to continue to report my observations and to complain when I saw no improvement. Innocently I assumed that no more than my initial outburst would be tolerated by the staff.

I presented to the world what I thought was expected of me: a rational, well disciplined woman, with only the slightest hint now and then that I was being subjected to anything out of the ordinary. My calm exterior was but a shell for the hurt and anger which lay beneath. "You're marvellous," my friends would say. "You're taking it so well. I don't know how you do it."

I would smile and tell them modestly that they would be exactly the same. "You have to be," I would say. "You have to be strong for the whole family ... It's quite natural, you know."

Because of course you couldn't possibly describe to them the inner turmoil which eats at you incessantly. Nor reveal the homicidal nightmare which plagues your nights, driving you insane; you dare not breathe a word lest they think you less than human. Nor could you bore them with how the whole dreadful thing was wrecking your life, your marriage – everything. They would have wondered what kind of a woman you were and whether you were after all really fit to be a mother.

- 0 -

The immediate crisis was over, and Andrew, although he no longer had a normal leg, was outwardly in one piece. Instead of bone there was metal, but the skin and flesh were still his own. We could all breathe again and we could rejoice.

Or could we?

The question of whether the leg would be saved or not had almost totally over-shadowed the real issue.

Had all traces of the cancer been eradicated?

Had the tumour, before its removal by surgery, allowed any of its corrupt cells to invade any other part of his body?

Had the chemo drugs killed off any stray cells which might have begun to wander, undetected?

Or had they caught it in time?

Nobody could answer these questions but we could not ignore

152

them. We could make calculated guesses, yes, but because statistics show two sets of results – the good and the bad – a lurking fear persisted that we might be wrong.

Statistics cannot be ignored, but I wonder if doctors have any idea which individuals will recover and which will succumb. Right from the beginning, had I been a doctor, I would have been tempted to put my money on Andrew.

But then I'm his mother. And more than anything else in the world, I wanted him to live.

- 0 -

A week later Andrew was transferred to the ward on the other side of the passage where patients were on the mend.

He quickly made friends with the others and greatly admired the famous aerobatics pilot in the end bed, Richard Goode, who had recently almost lost his life in a horrendous crash at an air display.

Andrew idolised him. He was not a big man, but even as he lay in his bed totally immobile you could tell by the expression on his face and the things he said that he possessed a huge, dynamic personality.

He became in Andrew's eyes a hero whose tragic injuries took on a far greater complexity than his own plight. Both his legs were multi-fractured, and although all the shattered pieces had been magically reassembled by Mr Sweetnam, the rumours in the ward were that he would never walk again without crutches, and certainly would never fly an aeroplane again.

"But he told me he *is* going to fly again, Mum. As soon as he's discharged. If he can then so can I."

This, I felt, was only wishful thinking.

'You have to have an A1 medical certificate to get a licence, Andrew,' I reminded him.

Yet Richard Goode provided a shining example to Andrew of how to deal with adversity. Later we heard that shortly after leaving hospital he did indeed fly an aeroplane again.

At the time, I failed to perceive how much this outstanding pilot's tenacity would influence Andrew. The cancer had dealt a catastrophic blow to his passionate dream to become a pilot, and even in the realms of a mother's fantasy I did not dare to hope that one day he too might be able to fly.

153

Chapter Sixteen

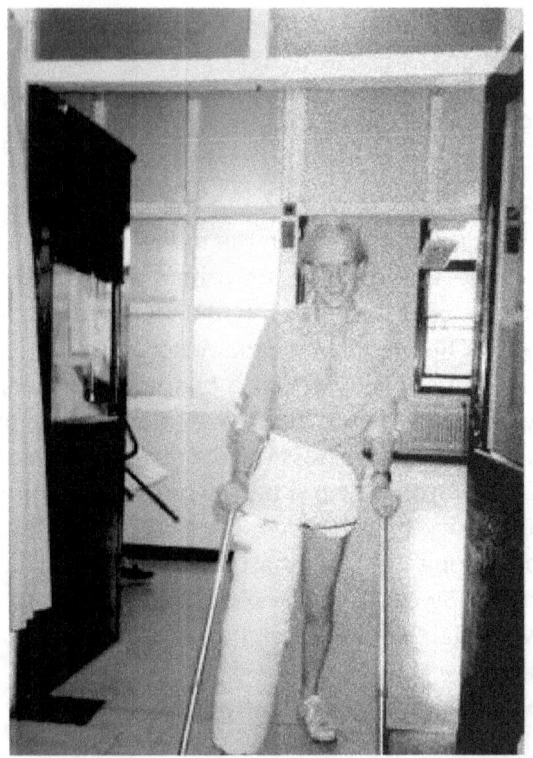

Great to be walking again – The Middlesex Hospital June 1984

Eight days after the operation Andrew took his first steps. What an exciting day it was! When we all trooped in that afternoon it was the main topic of conversation in the ward, and we were given a blow-by-blow description by the other patients who had urged Andrew on with enthusiastic encouragement and much hilarity.

"Come on, son," Colin said. "Let's see you do it again."

I held my breath and watched through mist-laden eyes as he teetered unsteadily across the room on the crutches, supported on either side by a physiotherapist and a nurse, laughing with the sheer exhilaration of his accomplishment.

Everything is relevant, I thought.

Quite soon he was able to walk up and down the passage, slowly and carefully though never without the help of a physio.

Once more Sister O'Leary laid down the law. "Don't even attempt to get out of bed unless a physio is with you, Andrew. And *never walk alone*."

Naturally he disobeyed these instructions.

With the typical idiot behaviour of an independent teenager he decided to go to the loo on his own. He slipped and fell heavily on his leg. A great cry of pain echoed through the whole of Dressmakers Ward, frightened everybody half to death and brought the nurses flying in from every direction to rescue him.

Sister O'Leary was furious. "*Andrew!* Mr Sweetnam would *kill* you if he knew!"

- 0 -

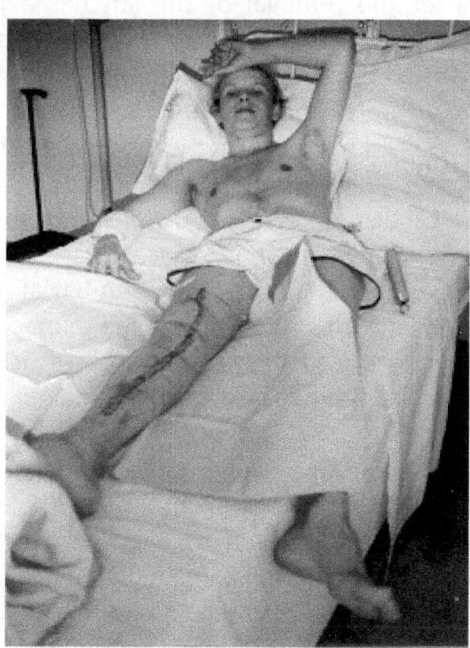

First sight of the 51 stitches waiting for a dressing

155

I was horrified at my first sight of Andrew's leg without the dressing.

"I just can't imagine it ever being right," I said in Colin's ear.

It was ten days after the operation. Sister O'Leary, a doctor, two nurses and a physiotherapist were gathered round the bed. The dressings had been removed and the fifty-one stitches taken out. Just before new dressings were applied, we were being permitted to see for the first time the long gash Mr Sweetnam's knife had carved down almost the whole length of the leg.

It looked terrible.

Purple, red and black, with some of the stitches looking very angry.

Colin gazed at this magnificent feat of modern surgery. "It'll take a while to settle down," he said philosophically. "Then all you'll see is the scar. It's amazing."

"It's also a strange shape," I whispered. "The leg seems to bend the wrong way."

It was twice its normal size, so swollen that you couldn't even see the contours of the new knee.

Immediately after the removal of the stitches a plaster of Paris back-cast was made which covered the entire leg but left a front opening so that it could be taken off for bathing and having the wound dressed. This cast, securely bandaged, had to be kept on for six weeks.

Sister O'Leary focused her steel blue eyes on the rebellious patient. "And during this time, Andrew, you must not bend the knee."

This was a surgical orthopaedic ward, which demanded the highest standards of nursing. Super efficient Sister O'Leary ruled it with a rod of iron, and at first Andrew did not get on with her at all well. She was impatient with his tantrums and threatened him on a number of occasions with banishment to the paediatric ward. It was much later that he said, laughingly, "Perhaps I should have taken her up on those offers!"

As the pain subsided he became more cheerful, but it was a student physiotherapist at the hospital who helped more than anyone else to achieve this. She had heard from her colleagues about a young man in Dressmakers Ward who came from Zambia. His name sounded vaguely familiar to her and when she came to see him they discovered to their delight that at the age of three they had been together at Parklands Nursery School in Kitwe, Zambia! They had not met since.

Her name was Nicola. She was not on his ward but made a point of visiting him several times a day, and by giving him constant support she slowly but surely took over the role Laura had earlier played.

They talked endlessly of all the things in Zambia which Andrew loved so much: the free and easy friendly atmosphere and the charm of the local people, the blue skies and sunshine, the swimming, the game parks, the mighty Victoria Falls – all the elements that had been part of his life and which he sometimes feared he would never see again.

I had a chat with Nicola one day. "You must miss Zambia," I said, having overheard some of their conversations.

There was a wistful look in her dark brown eyes. "I do," she said, flinging her thick rope of shiny black hair behind her back in a characteristic gesture which gave her an air of unstudied sophistication and assurance. "Very much indeed. But this is where I live now. So it's pointless to go on wanting to be in Zambia. My boy-friend would never get a job out there."

I felt my insides contract. Did Andrew know she had a boy-friend, I wondered, for I had a feeling he was becoming very attached to her. I had had an unfortunate encounter with Laura not long ago, which had given me a clear indication that their relationship would not last much longer. If this happened it would leave a serious void in Andrew's life which no doubt Nicola would have been a perfect candidate to fill. Although Laura and I had got on well, I had always been conscious of a restraint, more on her part than mine. Then one night shortly before Andrew's surgery she had spent the evening with him at the flat. We were in the kitchen making tea. Andrew was in the lounge watching television. She and Andrew may have had an argument but I noticed she was not her usual self. I had been about to say something when suddenly she turned on me.

"And you think you're so smart. So superior. You think I'm just dirt, don't you. You don't want me to associate with Andrew, do you? You don't think I'm good enough for your precious son. Well, let me tell you," she went on, not letting me get a word in edgeways, "Andrew and I would have made a go of it if it hadn't been for you, with your airs and graces. Just because you've got more money than I have doesn't make you any better, you know."

I was totally thrown off balance. Nothing could have been further from the truth and her words stung me to the quick.

"You're imagining it all," I said indignantly, suddenly certain she had

157

been bottling this up for a long time. "I'm very fond of you. I have never given you any cause to make you feel inferior. And why should I? I have the utmost respect for you. And I'm very grateful to you for all you've done for Andrew."

She had burst into tears then and the argument got nowhere. Afterwards I wondered if, because of my unnatural possessiveness for my son in his present state, I had subconsciously conveyed to her some resentment of his affection for her. Or maybe things had come to a head that night and she was just sad that it wasn't working out between them and she had to blame someone.

- 0 -

Colin Junior, who was still working as a mining engineer in Zambia, arrived in London en route to Menorca for his annual leave, and with Peter down from Manchester too, Andrew enjoyed having the whole family around him.

Young Colin adored his 'baby' brother and has always been very protective towards him, though because he is naturally not as demonstrative as Andrew, he doesn't show it outwardly. He sat next to Andrew's bed, squirming every time his young brother yelped with pain. He became cross with Andrew when he complained.

"Andrew," he said under his breath, "do you have to make such a fuss?"

"People have different levels of tolerance," I told Colin gently, sliding my arm around his waist. My sons were absolutely equal in my affection. I loved Colin dearly and had to be careful not to let him think I was favouring Andrew. "You could always withstand pain without flinching, even as a baby, because your pain threshold is naturally far higher than Andrew's. It isn't his fault."

Colin was also critical of the two cuddly teddy-bears that were always on Andrew's bed. As a child Colin had preferred toy fire-engines, trucks and cars to teddies. Maybe that was my fault. Maybe I didn't give him a teddy.

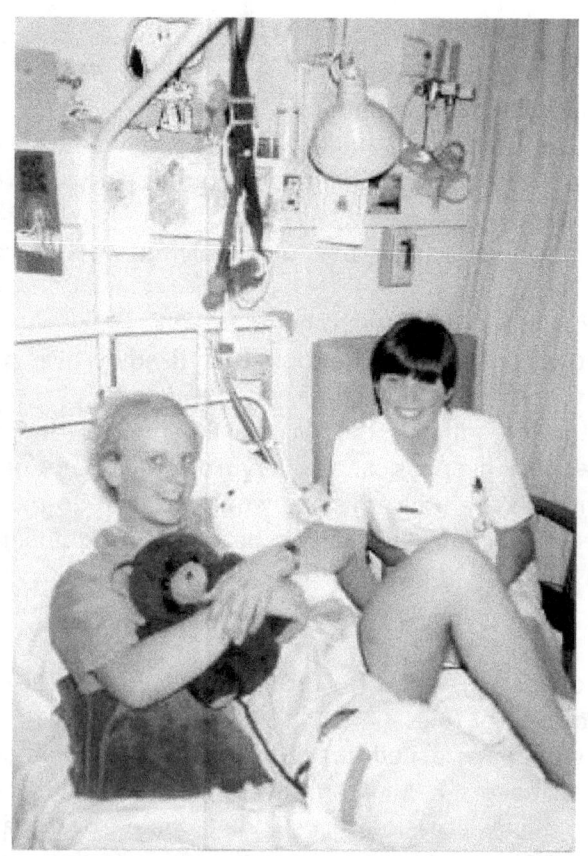

Andrew with his mascots, Dressmakers Ward,
The Middlesex Hospital, 1984.

"They're his mascots," I explained, smiling. "Given to him by various girl-friends to wish him luck. The brown one is called Rodney, after Mr Sweetnam. Isn't he cute? And the white one is called Laura."

- 0 -

Each day Andrew got stronger and was able to walk further and faster. The long period of recovery and rehabilitation had begun, and he was making excellent progress.

But alas. It would all too soon be halted, for there were still three chemotherapy treatments for him to endure.

159

"Do you know what day it is tomorrow, Mum?"

Grasping the triangular handle dangling over his head, he hoisted himself into a sitting position and reached for his diary.

I nodded, breathing in deeply as I searched my mind for something to change the subject. I knew, of course, only too well. But we had not discussed it.

"It's the first day of my fourth chemo."

He looked vacantly across the room then fixed his eyes on mine. He didn't need to tell me how much he was dreading it.

I had been dreading it too. We all knew that this one would inevitably set back his physical recovery from the operation, but none of us had any idea then that this one would hurl him to the edge of an abyss and leave him dangling in a void between life and death.

- 0 -

The pre-med was scheduled for three o'clock and Dr Mike would be putting the drip up at four.

Dr Mike was still attached to Greenhow Ward but had been a daily visitor to Dressmakers, helping Andrew to face the coming ordeal.

On one such occasion I couldn't help overhearing their conversation. "Why do I have to have this, Mike? I don't have cancer any more."

"Look, Boss, you know we can't stop now. We have to be sure so we have to complete the programme. Don't worry. I'll make certain it all goes without a hitch."

Three o'clock came and went. No pre-med.

Three-thirty.

Four.

No Mike and still no pre-med.

Andrew was extremely agitated and for the first time I defied Sister O'Leary's strict visiting hour rules. Andrew needed me and I stayed.

Half an hour later a strange doctor appeared at the bedside. No explanation, no smiles, but he had with him all the paraphernalia ready to put up the drip.

"But I haven't had my pre-med," Andrew protested. "And Dr Mike isn't here yet."

Andrew was appalled to hear that Mike was on an urgent case in Greenhow Ward. Instead, this skinny dark-haired iceberg, whom he had never seen before, was about to put up the drip. With horror I saw Andrew's strong resolve to withstand the treatment being totally undermined.

I stood up to my full five feet one and a half inches in front of the pushy doctor.

"Excuse me," I said. "He must have the pre-med before the drip can go up."

The doctor screwed up his face and looked at me as though I were mad.

I stared back at him. "Well, that's what always happens. Andrew is expecting it." A smile would go a long way too, I thought.

"And he has a fear of needles," I added, determined to put him in the picture.

"Absolute nonsense!" snapped the doctor, not an ounce of compassion in his eyes, no humour in his voice. Then he lifted his eyebrows. "Perhaps we should move him to a paediatric ward."

Andrew flinched, utterly crucified at being spoken down to like a small child.

I seethed with indignation. Why have they sent someone who clearly has no experience with sensitive teenage patients? Someone who seems to have been cast in a completely different mould to the rest of the caring doctors at The Middlesex? Someone with tunnel vision?

I wanted to tell him Andrew had needed a great deal of strength to prepare himself for this day. I wanted to tell him this effort had now been destroyed, but prudence stopped me and I said nothing more.

With his confidence in smithereens the state of Andrew's veins worsened. The whole exercise was extremely difficult and caused a great deal of pain and discomfort. It was an unjustifiable humiliation which made me purple with anger when I thought of all the dedicated care and attention Andrew had received from everybody over the long months of his treatment. From the ladies serving the meals. From the nurses. From the little green-eyed Sister, from Sister O'Leary, from all the junior doctors and the registrars. From Mr Sweetnam and Dr Jelliffe, Dr Annabel and Dr Mike, and countless others.

The friends who visited Andrew in the next few days found him either asleep or just too sick to respond. Six nurses from the private hospital he'd been in first, including Laura, came to see him, stood around his bed for a few minutes and left without him opening his eyes.

On Wednesday evening Brian Baverstock, Colin's oldest friend from his university days and his best man at our wedding, and his wife Grace arrived at St. Andrew's House. Colin Junior was still staying with us, and Brian drove us all to the hospital in time for the visiting hour.

- 0 -

On the dot of seven we tiptoe in. The ward is unusually quiet. Andrew is out cold. He is the only patient with a brown paper bag.

The five of us stand around the bed. There is a clinical smell. A mixture of Johnsons Baby Powder, Dettol and disease. The drip hangs over him like a clawing vampire, as though sucking the very life blood from his veins, the brown paper bag like a shroud.

His face is greyish white. The bones protrude, with sunken cheeks and deeply etched black circles round his eyes. A few wisps of white hair lie across his bumpy brow. His lips are dry and wrinkled.

He is motionless.

We stand looking down at him as though at a wake, in silent prayer, hands hanging down at our sides.

Finally we look up and with a nod from Colin we file out of the ward.

Our footsteps echo down the polished corridor leading to the swing doors at the end. I press the button for the lift. Staring at the blank magnolia walls, we wait silently for its shuddering arrival.

We walk out into the sunlight and cross diagonally over Mortimer Street towards the pub on the corner. Colin pushes open the swing door. He orders the drinks.

Grace, herself a retired nursing Sister, breaks the long silence. Her expression is one of undisguised horror.

"He looks dead," she says.

- 0 -

Andrew had no appetite, but every day he looked forward to the thermos of eight squeezed oranges I bought daily at the Leather Lane street market.

162

I loved the act of buying those oranges. I would walk up and down the colourful stalls, letting the sounds of laughter and shouting and music lift my spirits as I searched for the biggest, the shiniest, the firmest, the heaviest and the most orange of all the oranges. Collagen, which Vitamin C helps to create, plays an important part in the body's cellular stability, according to the foot therapy lady, and in its production of the hormones that help combat the effects of disease and surgery. I figured that with the major surgery Andrew had undergone, extra large doses would be needed, since clearly the more collagen his body produced, the faster the enormous wound would heal.

The staff at the hospital did not believe this theory.

"Okay," Dr Mike said when I cornered him one morning. "We'll write up the Vitamin E tablets you've brought in, but there is no clinical proof that Vitamin C makes any difference."

"What about all the other benefits of taking supplements of Vitamin C?" I asked.

Mike's eyes widened. "Like what?"

Still fresh in my mind, having been brought to my attention by the foot therapy lady, I recited them off like a parrot.

"First there's the feel-good factor. Less need for pain-killing drugs. A boost to the body's own natural immunity. A better appetite and a renewed sense of mental alertness ..."

He shook his head and I nearly gave up. "There's no proof," he insisted.

"But where's the proof that it does *not* help?" I retorted, going red in the face and aware of the unscientific question I had just asked.

Mike took my arm and led me to a chair in the passage, then sat down next to me.

"Osteosarcoma is one of the most vicious of all cancers and one of the most difficult to treat," he said gently. "There is no evidence whatsoever that Vitamin C can help."

I took a deep breath. "I have a child with a life-threatening disease. I cannot risk ignoring anything that might help, no matter how slim the chance. I know giant strides are being made in the treatment of osteosarcoma, especially here at The Middlesex. I know this but no treatment is ever guaranteed. Dr Jelliffe says fifteen percent don't make it. If your child had osteosarcoma wouldn't you think it was absolutely vital to do everything possible to augment the conventional aggressive treatment?"

Mike's face softened. I seemed to have hit a raw nerve. I pictured his new young wife. Perhaps a baby on the way.

"And you really think Vitamin C will help?" he said, his mind suddenly receptive. "What else do you think would help?"

It was typical of Dr Mike's generous nature that he was allowing me to have my say and I was not going to stop now. "A positive approach. An unwavering belief in Andrew's total recovery. Unrelenting support for him. And a sensible application of all known dietary aids in order to give his body its best possible chance. Don't you see, Mike? These are the only things that I have the power to control. Things I'm sure can all help to strengthen his immune system."

The foot therapy lady would be proud of me, I thought, as Mike's bleeper bleeped.

"In the case of osteosarcoma," I went on, certain I would never have another chance to speak my mind so freely to a doctor, "I know this holistic approach would never be sufficient on its own. But your conventional treatment, bolstered by any other approach which Andrew believes will benefit him, must surely have a better chance of success."

He stood up to go. "You know, I think you may be right," he said, and smiled. And only when he'd disappeared round the corner did I realise what the key words were in the whole of that conversation:

'... which Andrew believes will benefit him'

- 0 -

At the end of an interminable week the fourth chemo was over. The misery had now begun to show in Andrew's face. He didn't smile a lot and when he did he had lines that had not been there before.

He was eighteen but he looked three times that age.

"Smile, darling," I said when we visited him that evening. "Only two more sessions to go now. It's nearly over."

"How can I smile, Mum, when I feel so sick?"

I looked at Colin. "What is it Uncle Stan always says?"

"It's all right to smile and be cheerful
While life goes by like a song
But the man worthwhile
Is the man who can smile

164

When everything goes dead wrong."

Andrew roared with laughter, like he hadn't laughed for weeks.

I laughed too, and felt so much better for it. The foot therapy lady had said, "Laughing is the best emotional release valve we have," and I vowed that from then on I would try to cultivate more laughter between us all.

But the English A-level exams were due to start on Monday, and that was no laughing matter.

"Of course he'll be far too ill to take them," Sister O'Leary said as we stood discussing it in the passage, whispering so that Andrew would not hear her. "We're only allowing the arrangements to stand because it gives him something to work for and to look forward to."

Work on his set books had been almost impossible in such a busy hospital ward. He had listened to tapes whenever he could but the pain made it difficult to concentrate. In addition the past week of chemo had rendered him temporarily incapable of coherent thought.

Now there was only Saturday and Sunday left for him to recover.

"In any case," she said quietly, "he could never endure a three-hour paper. I would only agree if they were divided into two sessions, with three hours rest in between. We'll review the situation on Monday morning but you've seen for yourselves what he's like. His immune system has been attacked by the chemo drugs so right now his body's natural defences are extremely low. It will be out of the question."

- 0 -

In one way Sister O'Leary was right. Andrew was sick throughout the weekend. The pain, chemo drugs, sedatives, lack of food, incessant vomiting had all contributed to reducing him to a pitiful shadow of his former self, and the Shakespeare tapes stayed in their boxes.

I was appalled at how terrible he looked, how little energy he had. He just lay in his bed, pale, thin, weak and worn out. But even though his body had been physically attacked by the ruthless drugs fighting the cancer, his spirit had remained remarkably strong. It had never really wavered, and had been strengthened the moment the operation was over. I remember the feeling of exultation when he sat up in bed a few days after the surgery had been completed, and made an announcement:

"I now no longer have cancer," he had declared.

165

He had never before spoken about the cancer, only about the leg, and when he saw my surprised look he went on:

"They've cut it all out, Mum. It's gone forever."

This positive statement was the basis of his determined fight. Because he was so certain he not only gave his body the best possible chance of recovery, but gave it the best chance of reversing any spread of cells which may have escaped from the site of the tumour.

His total faith in Dr Jelliffe and Mr Sweetnam, backed by his family's belief in his recovery, had left him in no doubt that the treatment and the surgery he had received had resulted in total eradication of the cancer. If this positive attitude could be maintained I felt certain he would recover. This was great self-therapy for me too, and helped me to fight against those dreaded moments in the middle of the night when I couldn't get back to sleep and the doubt crept in like a cold draft from a window that wouldn't close.

Doctors cannot predict who will get well and who will not. They know that with this new treatment roughly fifteen percent will not get well, while eighty-five percent should recover.

Andrew had made up his mind he would be one of the eighty-five percent.

Besides, he had a dream.

He had a future to prepare for. A future as a pilot.

His A-levels were a vital necessity for that dream and for that future.

Nothing and nobody must stand in his way.

Chapter Seventeen

July 1984

On Monday morning a special room in The Middlesex Hospital Medical School was prepared for Andrew's A-level examination. The invigilator, one of the masters from Bradfield College, arrived early with the sealed papers.

Andrew woke feeling weak and sick. Nothing he ate or drank stayed down.

Sister O'Leary stood at his bedside, her face stern with authority.

"I'm sorry, Andrew, but we can't allow it."

"I don't care," he shouted, and struggled to reach for his crutches. "I'm going to do it! I must!"

Sister called Dr Mike.

"You're not well enough, Boss. And you'd be wasting your time. There's no way you can do it."

"Mike, I know I can do it. Please. Let me go!"

In the end they relented, shaking their heads as off he went in a wheel chair with the invigilator and a nurse who would be in constant attendance throughout the day.

Colin and I went back to St. Andrew's House and drank endless cups of tea.

"He must be feeling awful," I said, remembering how we'd held his retching body in the days following the first three treatments, and seen for ourselves how sick and debilitated and almost unhinged the drugs had left him.

"I'm glad he's giving it a go," Colin said. "But he'll never finish the paper. And even if he does he hasn't a hope in hell of passing."

But he did finish it, in spite of the vomiting, the dizziness, the headache, the pain and the state of utter exhaustion in which the chemo had left him – only more so this time because of the accumulative toxic effect.

That evening he looked up at us from his pillow and he grinned that

167

wonderful grin of his which no matter how skeletal his face, how pale and wrinkled his skin, how grey his countenance – still lit up his sunken eyebrowless eyes with an aliveness, a vibrancy we had seldom seen before.

"I did it!" he said, and my heart leapt into my chest just as it had all those years ago when he had finally conquered his brother's over-large bicycle.

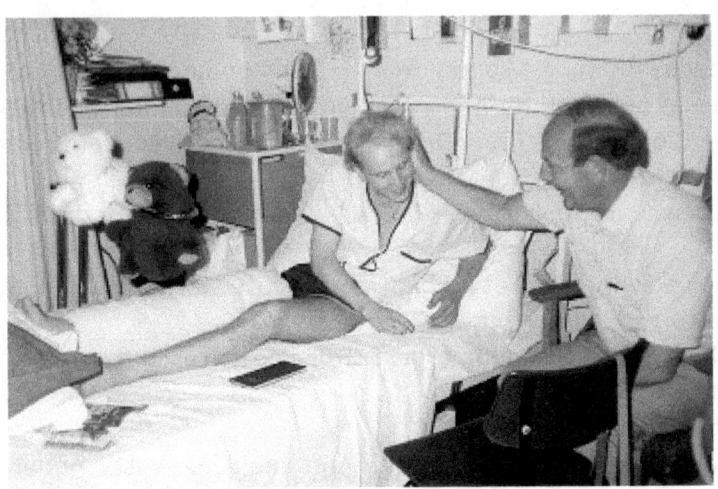

A word of praise from Dad

The next day Mr Sweetnam said he could start walking again. Good progress was made in spite of the week's set-back, so much so that the doctors unexpectedly decided to discharge him.

"I'm going home!" Andrew said, his voice singing with joy.

I was horrified. "It's far too soon," I said as we packed Andrew's clothes and stacked the piles of get-well cards into a plastic bag. "And how will we cope with the leg? He still has two English A-level papers to write!"

Nobody at the hospital gave us any advice about what to do or how to do it, but as usual when Colin was around, I needn't have worried. Back at St Andrew's House, in no time he worked out efficient systems for every aspect of the management of Andrew.

"We haven't even got a shower," I bleated to Colin after settling Andrew on the sofa with his English set books while we tried to make order out of chaos. "How are we going to bath him?"

Colin smiled. The kind of smile that epitomised his teasing contempt of my doubt that there were few practical things he could not solve. I should have known better, for a mining engineer is trained to solve everything from the extraction of the metal from the bowels of the earth, to the despatch of the finished product to the far corners of the world. "Not a problem," he said, and in the end the routine was worked out jointly by Andrew and his dad.

I stood in the bathroom doorway and held my breath. "Please be careful." I chewed my knuckles. "Mr Sweetnam will kill you if you bend the leg or jolt it."

First Andrew sat on a stool alongside the empty bath. Colin helped him in sideways, supporting the leg, then unwound the miles of bandages and removed the plaster cast, all in ultra slow-motion because any knock was excruciatingly painful.

"Okay. Let's fill the bath now," Colin said, turning on the taps luke-warm at first, watching Andrew's face as he gradually increased the heat.

At first Andrew needed a bit of help with washing though soon he could cope alone. Meanwhile Colin re-rolled the bandages, powdered the plaster cast and laid out the clean clothes in order of dressing. Luckily the weather was warm – the best English summer for many years – so Andrew could wear shorts.

When the bathing was finished the reverse process started: emptying the bath, drying, dressing the leg, putting the clothes on, then getting out of the bath sideways. Everything slowly and carefully so that the leg was not bumped.

Then, back on his crutches, he was ready for the day, the ablutions having taken just on an hour. Indeed I had worried for nothing.

- 0 -

The invigilator arrived at St. Andrew's House at nine-thirty on Thursday. Though still very weak and nauseous Andrew appeared full of confidence.

Colin and I left them in peace. In clear, warm July weather we wandered down Leather Lane, browsed around the stalls, bought the oranges and then stopped at a pub and sat at one of the tables in the sunshine. Drinking a beer and watching the fascinating stream of people thronging to and from the street market, we pretended to

169

enjoy ourselves.

"Stop worrying, Col. It's going to be all right. I promise you."

He pursed his lips. As the time was drawing nearer to his departure I had begun to see signs of the acute anguish he was suffering, that as a typical male he went to all costs to hide from everyone else. He wanted to be near Andrew all the time, just as I did, and it was tearing him apart that he had to leave so soon.

Colin could never talk when he was close to tears, and his silence emphasised my suspicions that he did not believe wholly in my optimism.

I took his hand in mine.

"Only by being quite sure ourselves can we hope to transmit our confidence to Andrew. You must believe that he will live. He will know if you don't."

We arrived back at the flat just as the exam was finishing. Andrew seemed quite calm, though exhausted. He wrote right up to the end of the three hours, which I thought was a good sign.

He had been sick only once.

The masters were taking it in turn to come up to London to invigilate, generously giving up their time to help Andrew. When Friday's paper was over everyone said how wonderful it was that he had done it. Now we would have to wait with fingers crossed until the end of August for the results.

Nobody thought that he would pass.

Colin shrugged. "Who cares? It's enough that he has done it at all."

- 0 -

On Saturday there is a sudden deterioration.

He looks terrible.

Paler and weaker than ever. A mouth full of ulcers which are so painful he can hardly swallow, let alone eat his breakfast. And a nasty looking open spot on the scar which today is angrier than ever.

Frantically Colin phones Dr Mike.

"Take him at once to St. Bartholomew's Hospital," Mike says. "Let them check him out there. It's only a stone's throw from your flat. Much quicker than coming all the way to The Middlesex."

Minutes later at the bleak Casualty Department at Barts Hospital the young, overworked Chinese doctor looks concerned.

"I think his count must be very low."

She fills a syringe and sends it for analysis.

The results are almost immediate. There is an anxious edge to her voice. "He must be re-admitted right now to The Middlesex, where they have all the details of his case."

She telephones Dr Mike. We thank her and help Andrew back into the car.

As we arrive home the phone rings. Colin picks it up. It is Dr Mike, speaking so urgently that when I put my ear as close to the phone as possible, I too can hear every word.

"Because of the very low blood count Andrew's condition is extremely dangerous. If he were exposed to any germs now he'd have no resistance whatsoever. His immune system has temporarily collapsed. The Adriamycin and Cisplatin have depressed the bone marrow, resulting in a decline of red cells which has led to anaemia. Also a decline of white cells which has lowered his defences against infection. There's a danger too that the depletion of platelets – vital for blood clotting – could lead to internal bleeding." He pauses. Then he says in what is almost a whisper:

"Anything which attacks his system now could kill him."

Colin and I look at each other in horror.

Mike continues in the same precise manner, making sure we understand every word he is saying. He is torn between having Andrew back in Greenhow Ward with possible exposure to germs, and leaving him at home with the danger of lack of on-the-spot medical attention.

"We'll compromise," he says. "We'll prepare a bed for Andrew right now. In twelve hours, if he's no worse, leave him at home. But if he gets any worse at all bring him in at once."

The twelve hours are like twenty-four. Colin and I pace the floor of the flat. We stare into space. We cannot believe that Andrew is now teetering on the edge of life and that one little germ could plunge him over the edge.

He does not get worse.

But when I look at his pinched grey face and his hunched shoulders and his mouth full of ulcers, I cannot see that he is any better either.

- O -

The suitcase was packed. The car taking Colin to Heathrow Airport was waiting in the forecourt.

Andrew clung to his father, tears flowing down his cheeks.

"Please come back soon, Dad."

Red-eyed, Andrew and I stood together in the doorway, stunned with sadness as we watched the car disappear out of sight, not knowing when we would see Colin again. I had been dreading his departure. I couldn't see how I would cope.

And I would miss him so much.

The weather was still gorgeous with clear blue skies, warm sunshine and no wind. Every day Andrew sat out on one of the benches in the forecourt. Laura came once or twice. We didn't see much of her any more, but there always seemed to be someone sitting on the bench with Andrew. Jo Rodin was a regular visitor and Nicola popped in every day. But oh, how we missed Colin.

Andrew still looked dreadful. Bent, bony and bald, he didn't seem to put on any weight and his clothes still drooped like a tragicomic clown's on his skeletal frame. Yet he was becoming stronger, and slowly the walking progressed.

The summer went on and on and gradually the sun tinged his pallid skin with a pinkish glow. Most of the time we stayed at St. Andrew's House, but now and again we took a taxi the couple of hundred yards to *The Old Mitre*, where Andrew's friends would gather to cheer him up.

He fought hard to maintain the moral strength he needed to keep going forwards. He had a goal. He had something important to live for, and though he never talked about his dream to be a pilot, I knew, as only a mother can know, that it was still foremost in his mind.

He loved life and this was all giving him an inner strength. And while his mind was boosting his body's own defences, gradually helping to replenish his suppressed bone marrow, I was attempting to feed him up to ensure he would have enough physical strength to withstand the next chemo treatment.

We lived from day to day. We became as close as ever a mother and son could be. I used this time to pass on to Andrew the wonderful gems of knowledge I was picking up from the meetings and lectures I attended from time to time – all stemming from my magical meeting with the foot therapy lady.

- 0 -

One evening Andrew cancelled a date with Nicola because he felt too ill to even go the short distance to *The Old Mitre*. When I could no longer bear the agony of watching him sitting in his chair writhing in pain, not even watching television, I felt I had to try to help him.

"You must relax, Andrew. The pain won't go if you sit there all tensed up. Come on, close your eyes, take a few deep breaths and just let everything go."

To my surprise he did just as I suggested. So remembering what I'd heard at a recent lecture about relaxation and mental imagery, I went through the steps with him, one by one.

"First tense all the muscles in your face, especially your jaw. Now imagine you can see this tension in your mind. Then relax the muscles. Can you feel the wave of relaxation? Okay. Now do this all the way down. One bit at a time. Neck, shoulders, arms, tummy, legs, feet. Until your whole body is floating on air. Close your eyes. First imagine you can see the tension. Then imagine you can see it melting into liquid jelly."

He opened his eyes and smiled. "That feels good, Mum."

"It'll feel even better if you can picture yourself in a beautiful place. How about the Luangwa Valley? You're sitting on the edge of the river, in the dappled shade of those lovely evergreen ebony trees. The Fish Eagle is making a plaintive noise, you know, a bit like the notes you sometimes make with your cello. The cicadas are droning their non-stop one-note chorus. The hippos are lolling in the river. You can hear the gentle swish of the water. There's a zebra just peering over the top of the long yellow grass –"

"Mum! You're making me homesick. But I see what you mean. It feels great."

"Okay. Now picture your white blood cells as an army. They've been training for weeks and they're ready to strike. Only you have to tell them where to go. You have to muster them, tell them to gather in a big group right in the middle of your chest, then WHAM! You tell them to strike."

He breathed in deeply and I was really excited to see that the imagery was working. "You know, Mum, I think I'll go to bed. It'll be easier to relax there."

I kissed him goodnight and thought what a good thing it was that like me he was so willing to try anything.

173

It was almost time for the fifth chemo treatment.
Neither of us had mentioned it.
We both dreaded it.

Chapter Eighteen

Greenhow Ward again, with its scrubbed floors and smiling nurses and ominous rows of brown paper bags.

First the blood test. The count must have been high enough for them to decide it was safe to proceed without giving him a blood transfusion first, but only just – in view of what happened afterwards.

He seemed perfectly content, so foolishly I went back to the flat. Soon after I arrived home the phone rang. I shuddered as I heard Andrew's voice.

"I just can't face it, Mum." He was sobbing, not sounding like Andrew at all. "I can't carry on. Please don't let them do it."

The room swam around me, walls, pictures and plants colliding in a Picasso of incongruous surrealism. I sat down, momentarily speechless.

Idiot! I told myself. *Why did you leave him alone?*

Andrew knew how easy it had become lately to manipulate me to suit his whims and fancies, but this was one time it would be fatal for that to happen. This was only the fifth treatment.

Six were necessary to save his life.

The words drummed in my head: *If he does not complete the treatment he will die.*

I had to answer him quickly. My first words would be vital. It would be so easy to say: *Darling I'll come right now and take you straight out of that nasty hospital ...*

Or I could say the right words to trigger his own innate strength to enable him to muster up enough will-power to carry on.

I panicked. What in hell's name were the right words?

"You must go through with it, Andrew," I said as calmly as I could. *If he does not complete the treatment he will die.* "I'll be there just as soon as I can. Don't worry, darling. Everything will be all right. You can do it."

Pretty pathetic words. Which of course he ignored.

"*No!* I want to get out. Now! I don't want any more of this."

I had failed hopelessly.

175

"Help me, Mum."

If he does not complete the treatment he will die ...

The words drummed into my skull ...

I kept on trying. "Please, Andrew. For your own sake. You must do it. I know you can do it."

But he was adamant, and when he put down the phone I felt sickened by my uselessness, my helplessness, my total inadequacy. I still had this unreasonable fear that I had done something wrong. I still felt it was my fault that he was so ill and now he was crying out for me to help him and I couldn't even do that. I desperately needed someone to guide me; I couldn't possibly go to him until I had the right formula to activate his own will to carry on.

What was wrong with me?

First I tried Peter in Manchester. If anyone could persuade Andrew it would be his brother, but after several phone calls to Andrew, Peter got nowhere either. I deliberately kept away from the hospital myself in the hope that the face-to-face appeals of others close to Andrew would be more successful, but after everyone had had a go – Jenny, Laura, Nicola, nurses, Sisters, doctors – he still would not budge.

All logical reasoning fell upon deaf ears.

Finally I tracked down Jo Rodin and plucked her from her busy schedule. After spending an hour with him she too failed.

But there was a chink in the armour.

When Jo gave up the struggle she came to see me at the flat.

She had one more card up her sleeve.

"Before you go to the hospital," she said, "I want you to phone Andrew once more. I want you to plead with him to carry on. If he still refuses, you must cry."

Cry?

This seemed all wrong to me. Jo had always told me I had to be strong. Now she was telling me to cry!

"Jo, I am not the crying kind. It isn't something you can turn on like a tap."

But she was not joking.

Fixing her penetrating blue eyes on mine she picked up the phone, dialled the number, asked for the phone to be wheeled to Andrew then thrust the receiver at me.

"Andrew, this isn't like you at all," I said quickly before I lost my nerve. "I don't know what's got into you. I want you to carry on. It's for your own good, darling. Let's stop this nonsense now."

"*Mum!*"

I hated what I was doing. I couldn't bear to hear the pain and despair in his voice. I wanted to save him but it seemed all wrong to force him to do something that was clearly too ghastly for him to contemplate.

"Help me, Mum. *Help me!*"

Jo sat opposite me, egging me on, urging me to cry. I was sure I couldn't do it, not just like that to order. But as Andrew went on and on and on I suddenly realised, *Oh my God! This is it. He is never going to give in.*

Only then, not because Jo had told me to cry but because I had no doubt now that it was hopeless, did I break into floods of tears.

At first Andrew was speechless. His mother, he must have thought, who had always been a rock of stability, was suddenly collapsing.

"*Mum!*" he yelled.

"I'm coming now, Andrew," I managed to whisper, and put down the phone.

Jo and I hurried to the hospital. Sister drew the curtains round the bed. Andrew and I held each other, both crying now; I because I knew he would die if he didn't have the treatment; he because he felt unable to endure it, but also because I was so visibly upset.

Suddenly he stopped crying.

His big sad eyes widened, the wrinkles around them and the deep dark circles beneath them making him look like the children I'd seen in a drought-stricken village in Zambia, who were dying of malnutrition.

The skeletal caverns of his face deepened. He held out his hands to me and I took them in mine, dreading his next words.

"Yes. All right!" he said, his body shaking with emotion. "I will do it. But I'm only doing it for you ... because I love you ..."

My mouth dropped open. I stared at his poor tired thin face, unaware at the time that he was doing this against all his physical and mental instincts and that this was the toughest decision he had ever made in his life.

Except that he didn't know then that it would be his tortured body that would make the final choice.

- 0 -

Although the decision was greeted with relief all round, the doctors decided that because the emotional upheaval had reduced him to a very low ebb he should go home for a few days and be re-admitted the following Monday. This seemed a good idea, though I was a bit doubtful and wondered with trepidation whether he might change his mind again by Monday.

It was a risk we would have to take.

I ordered a taxi. We held hands as it crawled towards High Holborn through the shimmering heat of London's West End. The streets were colourful with everyone in shirt sleeves and bright summer dresses. It was the eleventh of July, just a few days before the end of the school summer term. The final term of the final year of Andrew's schooling.

We had turned into Charterhouse Street and were just about to stop at St. Andrew's House when he leaned toward me and said, "Mum, wouldn't it be great if I could go back to school for the last few days of term?"

I looked at him with horror. "You must be crazy."

"Why not? It would be better than hanging around waiting to go back into hospital."

I took a deep breath. In his critically vulnerable state he could pick up any number of the germs that normally float around in boarding schools. I looked at his pale pinched face, his eyes so pathetically eager as he waited for the verdict.

I bit my lip. Oh, what the hell! If it was going to make him happy it was another risk worth taking.

- 0 -

He stayed with his housemaster and his wife this time, showered with kindness and care. He joined in most of the end-of-the-year festivities, and was thrilled to be awarded his House Colours. Delighted to have a little more time with Simon, Stuart and James before they all went their various ways into the world, this was indeed an unexpected bonus.

- 0 -

I was left in an emotional cesspool. I didn't want to see anyone, not even my close friends, and I was actually afraid to see people I didn't

178

know well; I hated it when for fear of hurting me or because they were embarrassed they were unable to say the simple words that would put us at ease with each other. I liked it when people said outright how sorry they were, even if they didn't mean it, or asked me how I was coping, rather than pretending that nothing was wrong at all. It made me feel as though they just didn't care.

Wearing my new soft wide flat unfashionable shoes it had taken me months to find, I walked for miles on my own, more and more often finding myself at the River Thames.

There is something special about that great wide ribbon of water that for me is the essence of London. Early in the morning with a misty haze over it, or at night when a myriad lights dance on its swiftly flowing surface, it never fails to thrill me. I love to stand on the bridges, and would often walk to the middle and stand gazing at the water, swirling and rushing and swishing as it has done for thousands of years. Hypnotised by the lulling movement I would think about Colin and my heart would ache with longing. Zambia was a million miles away: a misty pageant of jacaranda trees, vast blue skies and nights full of stars. A past life. A forgotten dream.

At night the other dream recurred. No matter how hard I tried to escape I was trapped in its all-enveloping mesh of glinting knives, laughter and blood.

- O -

After the precious few days back at school, Andrew got a lift home with a friend's father on Sunday when the term officially ended, and all too quickly it was Monday morning.

I had expected trouble at the last minute but when the taxi arrived he got in without a murmur. It looked as though everything would be fine.

- O -

Bed number one. In front of the nurses' station.

Blood test first. Old hat now but the count was much too low.

"Before we proceed he must have a transfusion of three pints," Dr Jelliffe said. "We will try to keep you almost totally anaesthetised throughout the treatment," he assured Andrew. "My registrar will do

179

all the preparation and will put up the drip himself."

I liked it. Having got this far nothing must go wrong and they were leaving nothing to chance.

A few hours after the start of the blood transfusion Andrew acquired a healthy looking glow, not seen since the chemo drugs began to deplete the red cells in his blood. The tea-lady cruising past with her trolley stopped and smiled.

"You look so well, luv!" she said, admiring his rosy cheeks.

I made it my special job to monitor the drip.

I watched the blood drip from the bag. Like a clock ticking. Drip drip drip. Down the plastic line attached to the cannula. Drip drip drip. Slowly into the tube. Drip drip drip. Into the vein. Drip drip drip ...

Twenty-four hours went by. The blood bottle was replaced by the first saline bag. The vein was showing signs of weakening so I kept an extra-steady eye on the apparatus to make sure it maintained a regular rhythm. Most of the time Andrew appeared to be out cold but struggled to open his eyes whenever anything new was about to happen.

On Wednesday I saw the first signs of unease. Please let nothing go wrong ...

I kept my eyes riveted to his face and miraculously the near-oblivious state was maintained. For him the world was blotted out and incredibly it all happened: the pre-med, the ice-cap, the cell-killing injection.

The brown paper bag went up.

- 0 -

Next morning I arrived extra early. Bleary eyed and taut with tension I continued my vigil. The curtains were kept drawn around the bed, the two of us cocooned in the mock privacy except for the frequent popping in of nurses and doctors.

Then little by little I sensed him becoming restless.

Suddenly the drip stopped.

I yanked open the curtains and shouted.

"Nurse! Come quickly!"

She rushed in, adjusted the drip, but I could still see that the vein, weakened by the non-stop inflow of fluids since Monday morning, was in a bad way.

I suppose I could have predicted the chemo treatment would fail that afternoon. Nothing was right, really. He was restless. He vomited every time he woke up. He was nine-tenths unconscious yet inexplicably conscious whenever threatened. The drip wasn't going in properly.

And then, for some extraordinary reason, the registrar disappeared and there was another change of doctor.

Three o'clock. The pre-med. So far, so good. If we can just get through today I know it will be fine, I tell myself.

Three-fifteen. The drip plays up again. I adjust it – an expert now – twiddling the button on the side of the valve below the drip bag as I've seen the nurses do.

Three-twenty. The drip is even more erratic.

Three-thirty and they're trying to put the ice-cap on his head.

Suddenly he opens his eyes.

"Please, please don't start anything till I'm asleep –"

In his semi-conscious state he moans and twists his head as he fights the instrument of torture. But they keep trying. Stubborn idiots, I think to myself.

But this time I say nothing. The distraught nurses are striving to do their best but it just isn't working.

Finally they give up.

"We'll leave him for a while," the little green-eyed Sister says as the nurse carts away the ice-cap. "See if he'll calm down a bit."

I sit close to him and watch. He looks unconscious but opens his eyes whenever he feels insecure.

Ten minutes later they bring in the ice-cap and try again.

"No! Please don't do it till I'm asleep ..."

"Leave it!" I say fiercely. "It won't make any difference anyway."

They stop, but not before the carefully calculated state of semi-consciousness has been broken. An unforgivable setback in my opinion for the sake of a few wisps of already dead hair.

"Please don't start anything till I'm asleep," he murmurs again and again, his voice tailing off until it is almost inaudible. "Please ... please don't start anything till I'm asleep ..."

- 0 -

The doctor creeps in through the screens, syringe poised.

"I don't think the drip is working properly," I whisper urgently. "It keeps stopping and it's very irregular."

She nods, waits a few moments, then decides to get the injection over as quickly as possible before Andrew wakes up again.

She pushes the plunger down and the thick red invasion of killing metals begins to enter the vein.

Suddenly the arm begins to swell. She jerks the needle out and fiddles with the drip. Sister rushes in. Then the nurses. They send for the Registrar who calls Dr Jelliffe. He looks at Andrew, then at my distraught face.

"The arm can no longer sustain the drip," he tells me gravely. "The vein has started to leak again. It will be dangerous if the drugs are allowed access to the body by any other route."

The glaze clears from Andrew's eyes. He is wide awake now, his expression like one possessed – furious, frantic, frenzied ...

I watch, open mouthed, my heart thumping, my body in a cold sweat.

Surely they are not stopping altogether?

They must carry on!

But nothing happens. After a week of hoping and praying and wishing and wondering if it will be successfully completed, the treatment is suddenly abandoned!

"But it's not complete," I argue.

My well-disciplined exterior cracks. I plead with them. I argue. I shout. I quote Dr Jelliffe's statistics: "Eighty-five percent survive if they have this new treatment. Fifteen percent don't. Six treatments are necessary for Andrew to survive and he has only had four and now a tiny bit of the fifth! How can you stop now?"

Suddenly I am the patient. They calm me down with cups of tea. The Sister talks to me, then the doctor, then the registrar. And finally Dr Jelliffe.

"The signs are loud and clear," he says, calling me aside. "Both physically and mentally the point of saturation has been reached. To go any further could be fatal."

182

Right now, in this hospital, he tells me, there is a boy a bit younger than Andrew who has received too much chemo and has gone into an irreversible toxic state.

I swallow hard. I think I am beginning to understand.

"You mean –"

Dr Jelliffe nods. He says, quietly, "There is nothing more we can do."

Slowly, like a cockroach crawling up my spine, it begins to dawn on me. They are not only stopping today's chemo and tomorrow's. They are stopping the whole goddam programme. It is finished. All over.

They are stopping because to carry on could kill him.

All along I had thought that not to carry on would kill him.

- 0 -

It was only the next day that I fully understood.

"People react in many different ways to chemotherapy," Dr Jelliffe said patiently, having sat me down opposite him once again in the quietness of his consulting room. "The tolerance level is extremely varied. Some take it in their stride. Others find it unbearable. Their reactions cannot be predicted. The dosage we give, although scientifically calculated for each individual case based on the careful study of previous cases, the kind of tumour it is and how far it has spread, is in the end always a calculated guess and there are bound to be some who get too much. Or not enough."

Little by little it grew clearer.

"Last week," he said, "when Andrew said he couldn't take any more, his condition was already perilously low and his body had probably reached the limit of its tolerance then. Drugs which produce very severe vomiting were sometimes used as a means of torture in war and espionage, as a method of totally breaking a captive and causing complete submission. Andrew was reacting, or rather his body was reacting defensively against the ultimate state of submission. He was fighting it without knowing why he was fighting it but just because he knew he could not take any more."

Dr Jelliffe reminded me that the new treatment was still in an experimental stage and they were trying to refine it all the time. (One of the most significant advances in chemotherapy treatment today is the vastly increased tolerance of the drugs by patients. They have

183

come a long way.)

"It may well be that some patients need less than others," he went on. "Some may recover without any chemo at all. Some will die anyway. We look at each patient as an individual. This one may need six treatments or maybe seven. This one only three. We don't know ..."

I smiled at Dr Jelliffe, understanding at last. I told him it would be nice to think that as new horizons are explored the eighty-five percent survival rate might one day be overtaken by yet a higher percentage, perhaps influenced by lessons learned while treating Andrew.

That night on the phone to Zambia I quelled Colin's shock and consternation by telling him that Dr Jelliffe had said that completing the planned six treatments could only have made about two percent difference to Andrew's chances of survival.

- 0 -

And so it was over. The equipment was wheeled out and Andrew was left to sleep off the sedatives he'd been given.

In a state of emotional shock I ran down the stairs to meet Mick, an old friend from Zambia who was in London for a few days on business. He had called at the hospital several times during the day and had said he would pick me up at seven-thirty to take me out for dinner. He was still waiting in the entrance hall at nine-thirty.

I almost didn't see him and he almost didn't see me; I was exhausted and with my long hair awry and make-up non-existent I knew I looked a mess. He took me to the Founders Arms on the South Bank because he knew I loved the Thames. We sat next to the window where I could look out at the river with its ripples of silver and floodlit St Paul's Cathedral majestic in the background. Over dinner and a bottle of wine he listened while I poured out the events of the week. I don't think he will ever know that he kept me sane that night.

- 0 -

The next morning as I hobbled up Berners Street towards The Middlesex I watched the sun glint on the Post Office Tower, lighting it up like the beacon of hope I was now convinced it was.

While I packed Andrew's bag, the little green-eyed Sister took both his hands in hers. "Good luck, Andrew," she said in her kind, soft voice.

184

"And phone me if ever you need help."

Weak and unsteady on his crutches he went to each bed to say goodbye to the old men in the ward and offer a few encouraging words. Sister walked with us to the door. Andrew turned and waved. He was leaving Greenhow Ward for the last time, and his face was a strange mixture of sadness and euphoria.

In the taxi he sat back.

He saw me looking at him and his thin face puckered into a wrinkled smile.

"Well, they've all done their bit, Mum. Now I reckon it's my turn."

Chapter Nineteen

June 1999

Dear Andrew,

When you asked me what I remember after all these years about when you first told us you had cancer – very little. 'Cancer' then was only a word. I'd had no experience of cancer, no experience of anyone dying or being really ill. I was very young and not very conscious. So it was a slow reaction really. Of course I didn't know then what lifelong consequences meant and I still struggle with that one.

Well, there we are. But I hope some of this will help to fill in the picture for you.

I remember being down Old Study Passage and you had a lot of pain from being hit in your leg with a hockey stick or a ball. It seemed that it should have been just a bruise but it hung around for a long time and you were in agony if it got knocked. You went to the San but they had no answer and thought you were making a fuss. Then I remember you had taken yourself off to a specialist because you weren't happy with the school doctor's apparent lack of concern.

I don't remember you actually telling me you had cancer at that time and it wasn't until we came to see you in hospital that the reality dawned on me or any of us really. I never thought that you wouldn't make it. I was sure the doctors would fix it and didn't really worry. So after seeing you in hospital it all became real. Because before, when you weren't at school, we could only imagine what you were experiencing.

I remember your room when you came back, and the atmosphere in the room. It was a very emotional time, seeing you looking so different. Your appearance hadn't really changed except for your hair and the loss of weight, but something inside you had. And the fear. You were so frightened.

One thing that has always stuck in my mind was when you told me you were faced with having your leg taken off. That was really shocking and very upsetting.

Before we went to the hospital to see you we weren't involved. We were concerned but didn't understand really. Cancer was something other people had and died from. So I couldn't believe you had cancer, not at that age and not from being hit in the leg. So it wasn't real. But seeing you, seeing your eyes, the tears in them, it was horrible. It was really happening and you could lose your leg and this could have happened to me or Stuart.

Stuart and I were shocked and we both sat around together feeling very worried and like a black cloud over us. We did not stop thinking about you and were always anxious to hear how you were doing. We were always talking to the house-master. It was acknowledged that the three of us were very good friends. I think we must have had a chat about you coming back to school with the housemaster.

I remember bathing you the last time you came back. It was then that I understood what they had done to you, your bandaged leg propped out of the water and seeing how weak you were and the effect of the chemo and losing your hair.

You were quite helpless really and I realised then what

you had gone through at the hospital which the flowers, cards, smiling well-wishers and clean sheets had done a good job of concealing. Things like how you had gone to the loo. All things that make my hair stand on end.

I really admired your courage and strength in dealing with all that you did. You were very brave. I don't think I could have coped like you did. It was very moving, very humbling giving you a bath. It made one think of old people needing care, taken to the loo etc. and what they must think having young nurses and carers looking after them.

I remember Stuart and I struggling to keep a brave face in case you saw in our faces what we really felt. That was hard. We wanted to keep your spirits up and keep you going.

What I found very tragic was the consequences for you with the flying. You could never be a pilot now. One of Life's really cruel blows.

Or wasn't it meant to be? Who knows?

Love, Simon

Chapter Twenty

July – November 1984

I watched Andrew come out of the darkness of the last six months.

No one knew what would happen. No one knew how many peaks and valleys he would still have to traverse, or how hazardous they would be.

No one knew yet whether his new leg would survive.

Or whether he would live or die.

It was the beginning of his own personal battle. The beginning of a new life. A different life. There was so much to accomplish. So much to learn. Until now he had been plastic in their hands, responding passively to their medical manipulation. Now it was up to him alone to make things happen.

To sing his own song.

To live.

- 0 -

First he had to learn how to bend the new knee, how to walk and re-educate his muscles and all the plastic bits. The leg had become stick-like, weak and useless.

He had lost thirty pounds in weight.

The first stage was daily physiotherapy at The Middlesex. Transport was going to be a problem. I could have done with a car but parking would have been a nightmare. We managed initially with taxis until sensible Nicola, who met Andrew every day at physio in a proprietorial way, took matters into her own hands.

"You know, Andrew," she said one morning when we stood waiting for a taxi, "there's no reason why you shouldn't travel on the Underground."

"Nicola!" I said, imagining him slipping and falling and smashing the delicately constructed new leg. "It's out of the question."

189

"It's okay," she said. "I'll go with him the first time if you like. To re-initiate him."

Nicola won. She also banned me from that first journey.

It was a real breakthrough. Now he had independence and freedom, and he became once more the possessor of a weekly London Transport pass. I still have that pass. I cry inside whenever I look at the hollow eyes in the pinched, hairless face and remember his stoic determination and his courage.

The physio sessions were the highlight of his day. He worked feverishly hard at the exercises, and the sessions in the hydro-pool not only began to put muscle on his new leg but strengthened his whole body.

In one way Nicola had imperceptibly taken over from Laura. Though not officially on his case she gave him great encouragement, bullying him and instructing him with an authority way beyond her years to 'keep your bottom in ... straighten your back ... keep your shoulders level!' They became really good friends. She often visited him at the flat and sometimes took him to *The Old Mitre*.

One night, tired of cooking, I suggested we go for a meal at the Founders Arms on the South Bank. We couldn't get a taxi back for love nor money. "We can walk," Nicola said, as though this was the most natural thing to do, "and maybe pick up a taxi on the way," she added when she saw my look of horror.

We ended up trudging all the way down Hopton Street, Southwark Street, and then on to Blackfriars Bridge where eventually we found a taxi – a marathon walk for Andrew and every step an agony of endurance.

At the end of the first four weeks of physio it was time to think about leaving London and establishing our base at our own flat in Manchester. Besides, there was Peter and Andrea's wedding on the eighteenth of August. Mr Sweetnam gave Andrew the go-ahead to register at a hospital not far from our flat in south Manchester, which he said had a new physiotherapy department second to none.

Colin arrived from Zambia on a hot Monday morning in the middle of August, packed up the London flat, piled all the plants and pictures I had bought into a hired four-by-four and drove us up to Manchester.

The wedding was in north Wales amongst the hills and the valleys and the gurgling mountain streams. It was a joyous occasion, a wonderful relief from the tension and strain of the past seven months.

Andrea was radiant in a fairy-tale dress with a full length veil, and with Peter in a grey morning suit and top hat they made a handsome couple. I had bought Andrew a new dove grey suit off the peg, hoping it would fit because all his other clothes hung on him as though they belonged to someone twice his size.

I was lucky. It fitted him perfectly.

Colin Junior and his wife Heather were on leave specially for the wedding, and Philip and Jo were there too, to share our pleasure. So was our very dear Jesuit friend from our Williamson Diamonds days in Tanzania: Father George, lover of people, literature and music, who had flown from New York to participate in the service. Oh, how good it was to have his blessing, and how good it was for the family to be together, to relax and to be happy.

But every time I glimpsed Andrew's gaunt face, with the dark-rimmed sunken eyes and the wisps of dull white straw still clinging to the bald head, and the new grey suit drooping from the skeletal shoulders, a sadness filled my heart which not even the merriment and happiness of the wedding could dispel.

Would he recover, I asked myself as I sipped my champagne? And if he did, would he ever be in the position Peter was in today? Would he ever appear at the door of a church, a radiant bride on his arm, smiling at her and she smiling at him, covered in confetti and posing for the cameras? I wanted so much for him to be happy. Laura had gone out of his life, and now Nicola was far away in London. He was so full of love and he needed someone to love, but looking as he did, would any girl ever want to spend the rest of her life with him?

I couldn't bear the thought of this not happening.

Andrew had said he was determined he would dance at Peter's wedding. We had all smiled, knowing this would be impossible. A few minutes after the bridal couple had circled the floor I couldn't believe my eyes when I saw him on the floor too, propped up by one of the bridesmaids. You could hardly call it dancing, but when he sat down, exhausted after shuffling only half a circuit on the floor, he looked at us and grinned.

"I did it, Dad! I danced!"

On Sunday the happy couple flew to Zambia for their honeymoon, travelling with Colin Junior and Heather who were returning home to Kitwe after their long leave. They were all going to the Luangwa Valley, to one of the most beautiful and prolific game parks in the whole of the continent of Africa, at the best time of the year for viewing game: at the end of the dry season when the grass was short and water scarce.

In the car driving back to Manchester after the wedding, Andrew was sullen and silent.

"What's wrong?" I asked him, wondering if it had all been too much, too soon.

He tapped me on the shoulder and pointed to his head.

Only then did I notice that the last of his wispy white hair had gone, leaving his head shiny and smooth and bare.

"It fell out in the bath this morning, Mum."

I took his hand and squeezed it. "Well," I said, trying not to sound too flippant, "you were very clever to make it stay just long enough for the wedding photographs!"

But it was the complete loss of body hair that upset him most. He hated the unmasculine smoothness: the hairless limbs, the naked chest, the lack of pubic hair. I expect that after months of being treated like a child, watched over and protected by everyone, it was all part of his desire – his need – to be a man.

A few days later he went back to London for a check-up with Mr Sweetnam and Dr Jelliffe.

"Well, everything is fine, Andrew," the doctors all said, pleased with their handiwork. "Come back and see us in two and a half months' time."

- 0 -

The A-level results were due shortly. We had chosen not to speak about them at all, certain that having been written under such horrendous conditions there was no chance whatsoever that he could pass.

When the school phoned with the results Andrew was ecstatic.

He blinked his eyes and shook his head and a smile spread all over his face. "This is unbelievable! I gave it everything I had but I never thought I'd make it."

Colin was almost speechless. "Congratulations, son," he managed to say. "It does you credit."

I gave him a hug. "You did it in spite of that pig of a master who said on your report that beach boys don't pass A-levels."

192

"Sometimes masters like that can bring out the best in you," Colin said, laughing.

I smiled back my tears of happiness. "What is it we always say? Nothing ventured, nothing gained."

"That's for sure, Mum. But I'd better hurry up and get at least one more A-level." And straight away he grabbed the Yellow Pages to look for Sixth Form colleges in the Manchester area.

His success was a much needed boost to his confidence, and eager to make up for lost ground he decided to enrol immediately at St John's College in the city centre to do A-level Law.

"Good idea," Colin said. "You could set up in partnership with Peter."

Andrew shrugged. I could see his mind churning around his lost flying career. He sighed. "Peter said it would be a useful A-level to have. He said even if I didn't make it to University to read Law I could at least be a Barrister's clerk."

"It's too soon for him to be thrown into the world of normality," I told Colin that night. "Look how weak he still is. Even with his crutches he's unsteady. He'll be entering a totally new world, strange and unfamiliar after the cloistered existence he led at Bradfield College. We should stop him."

"You try to stop him," Colin said. "I won't. He's made up his mind."

- 0 -

The next day, as we stood in the long queue of boisterous students from every walk of life my heart broke as I stared at the back of my son's shiny bald head. He looked so out of place, an outcast in this motley crowd of healthy, robust youngsters waiting to enrol. Yet later he assured me that everyone had been friendly.

"They were great, Mum. They all treated me perfectly normally."

I wondered if this was all part of Andrew's need to be normal, his determination to be just like everyone else, but at the time there was only one person in his class whose demonstration of friendship seemed to have any meaning for him.

Her name was Julie.

A young girl who appeared quite undeterred by his appearance. Slim, with soft dark curls framing her oval face, she had the bluest eyes I had ever seen. More importantly she was gentle and kind.

193

And Andrew adored her.

I was happy to see him with such a lovely girl but I was terribly afraid for him. I didn't want him to get too fond of her; I couldn't bear to think of him being hurt, so I didn't actively encourage the relationship.

- 0 -

Andrew's nineteenth birthday fell on a warm sunny Sunday just before Colin had to fly back to Lusaka. Friends and family gathered. We sat out in the garden, soaking up the September sun, listening to the sweet melodic tunes of the blackbirds and breathing in the soft earthy smells of approaching autumn. Andrew cut his cake and blew out his candles while we sang 'Happy Birthday' and pretended that everything was normal.

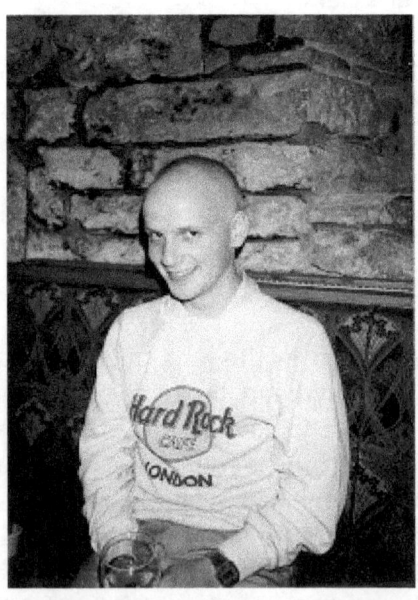

No other birthday in our family has ever stirred such poignant feelings. Birthdays are usually celebrated without giving much thought to the meaning of the celebration, but we were rejoicing in this one because so far, he was alive.

Colin and I looked at each other as we raised our champagne glasses to those who had made this possible.

194

"Here's to Philip and Jo," Colin said.

"And Dr Jelliffe and Mr Sweetnam," I said, clinking my glass all round the table.

"And to all the other doctors and nurses at The Middlesex Hospital," said Andrew, who was drinking Coke in a wine glass because the chemo had resulted in his total abhorrence of alcohol.

He was nineteen.

He was alive.

Neither his baldness, his thinness nor his lameness stopped him from being happy that he was alive.

"Life is sweet," he said.

Nostalgically we remembered my father. He had stayed with us in Zambia while recovering from his second leg amputation due to a circulatory illness. He loved sitting on the patio in his wheelchair sipping his sun-downer sherry and watching the mango trees at the bottom of the garden silhouetted against the vast flaming African sky as the sun plunged into the distant bush. One evening a friend had joined us.

"Dr Taylor, how do you manage so well with no legs?"

My father looked at us all with those pale blue piercing eyes of his and smiled.

"Life is sweet," he said, with an added twinkle in his eye.

After that it had always been difficult for us to complain about anything.

- 0 -

At Manchester Airport Andrew and I said our tearful farewells to Colin. We were on our own again. Not really alone because we had Peter and Andrea who had bought a house near our flat, and we had Colin's elder brother Stan, who automatically took Andrew under his wing.

Stan's hobby was rifle shooting. He shot for Lancashire and encouraged Andrew to follow in his footsteps – a sport where you didn't have to walk or run. Andrew had been an excellent shot at school and was keen to pick it up again. They went every Monday and Wednesday to the rifle club and soon Andrew was showing such promise that Uncle Stan wanted to enter him in a big competition at Blackpool.

For this he would need his own rifle, but first he had to apply for a

195

licence. With unusual compassion the local friendly policeman dealing with the application said he would make a special effort to expedite it. He understood that target shooting was all Andrew had to replace the golf, hockey and squash he had so loved.

It was not only the policeman who showed compassion. Andrew's youth, his crutches, his pale face and his bald head drew glances of curiosity and pity from strangers and provoked concern, sympathy and admiration from friends.

But it could also have the opposite effect.

One night to give Andrew a change of scenery we went to a quiet, smoke-free pub down the road, close enough for Andrew to walk. He tired very quickly and since he didn't like alcohol he decided to walk home on his own while we finished our drinks.

When we arrived home we found him sitting on the sofa with his head in his hands, obviously very upset.

I sat down next to him. "What's wrong?" I asked, my hand on his arm.

He shook his head. "I still can't believe it. I was walking towards the traffic lights. So I could cross where it was safe. There was this girl. Walking just in front of me. A young girl. About my age. She must have heard the clunk-clunk of my crutches on the pavement. She turned round. Took one look at me and started running!"

I had a mental picture of the girl turning and seeing the bald head and the combat jacket a friend's son in the army had given Andrew and I could understand her fear.

"I kept going. Didn't walk any faster or any slower. The lights were green but she was obviously terrified and kept looking over her shoulder. Suddenly she disappeared into the driveway of the doctor's surgery next door to our flat. She hid in the shadows while I clunked past. As soon as I went through our gate she darted out and fled down the road, her long hair flying and her handbag flapping. It was awful, Mum."

I went to the kitchen and made him a mug of hot chocolate. "Forget it, Andrew. What she saw had nothing to do with you, personally. The things that frightened her were only outward things. The combat jacket. The crutches. Your bald head ..."

I did wonder about the fondness he had for that combat jacket. Because he knew now that he would never be able to join the RAF, he seemed to attach a kind of sentimental value to this jacket given to

196

him by someone who was achieving his own goals in the British Army.

Then a few nights later he went to another pub to meet some old friends. He knew one of the part-time barmaids there, a Law student. When the landlord saw her talking to Andrew he said, "I want that skin-head out of here!"

Andrew heard him, and although the man was apologetic when she explained about the cancer, Andrew was very upset.

Not that he wanted sympathy. On the contrary, he wanted to be treated exactly like everyone else.

It was difficult for *me* to do this. I 'mothered' him too much, but how could I do otherwise? He needed looking after.

I knew, of course, that I would soon have to leave him to get on with life by himself. He was nineteen and he needed his freedom. But I could not go yet. He still had his ups and downs. More ups than downs, but when he had nightmares, when he felt his life was in pieces and he was unable to face the future, he needed me there to shout at and vent his anger on. Every set-back depressed him. His moods swung between elation and dejection, though the bad moods were popping up less and less frequently.

There were also many days when he didn't feel well, and he was nearly always tired. Sometimes at night he would look at the food I had prepared. "I'm sorry, Mum. I don't feel like eating. I'm just too tired. I think I'll go to bed."

To prepare him for the future I taught him which foods were best for him and how to cook them. Plenty of fruit and vegetables. Plenty of fibre. Avoid too much fat, salt, or sugar. Not too much meat, coffee or tea, but drink Rooibos tea which has no caffeine and very little tannin. A daily glass of fresh orange and extra high doses of Vitamin C supplements, so important for the stability of the cells, regardless of what the doctors say. And no junk food.

Yet even when he wasn't feeling well, or when it was very cold and wet, he forced himself out of bed and went to College. And every afternoon he went to the hospital for physiotherapy.

- 0 -

After several weeks, when Andrew was well established in his routine, I suddenly reached a stage of unprecedented physical and mental exhaustion. It came upon me completely without warning and even I

197

recognised I was near to breaking point.

Peter came to see me. "Go back to Zambia, Mum. Go home to Dad."

"I can't leave Andrew yet. You know that."

Peter compromised. "Okay, go to Menorca for two weeks. Only one thousand miles away instead of five. It'll be good for Andrew to have a trial period on his own."

To me even this was unthinkable. I struggled with my conscience. It was bad enough that I had left Colin on his own all these months but out of the question that I should now abandon Andrew too; yet I recognised I had to do something or I would become ill. The dream had suddenly returned after some weeks of peace, this time assuming a new, gorier form. It also lasted longer and I would wake up with the horror still all around me as though it were real.

Reluctantly I bought a ticket for a Dan Air flight to Menorca. I filled the fridge and freezer and convinced myself Andrew would have everything he needed.

Peter dropped me at Manchester Airport on his way to work. As though in a trance I handed over my ticket at the Dan Air desk, wandered through the main hall with its double row of giant chandeliers, bought a glossy magazine from W H Smith's, and took a seat to wait for the call to board the plane.

I looked around at the sea of holiday makers in their brightly coloured track suits and shiny shorts. What on earth am I doing here? I don't *want* to go to Menorca. I want to be with Andrew. He needs me ...

I sleep-walked to the barrier and showed my boarding pass.

I felt a tightness in my chest. I was beyond the point of no return, locked in a one-way tunnel with the only exit leading to an aeroplane that would whisk me away to my Mediterranean retreat.

I was running away!

Why?

I didn't want to run away.

I looked around for a phone. I would call Peter. Tell him to come and fetch me. That I had never intended to go. That this was all a hideous mistake.

I groped in my handbag for ten pence pieces. Dialled Peter's number.

Blurted out my fears.

198

"Don't be silly, Mum. Andrew will be fine. Just you go and enjoy yourself."

Enjoy myself!

I heard his placid voice, his level-headed, practical words. I didn't have the strength to argue any more.

Like a lemming I shuffled with the other passengers into the plane, unable to turn back. I fastened my seat-belt. If anything happened to Andrew I would never forgive myself.

I stared at the clouds all the way to Menorca, thinking about him.

Oh, yes. He looks so unafraid. He seems so content. He acts so normally, just as his grandpa always did, that often I think there is nothing wrong with him at all. As far as he is concerned, there is not anything wrong with him. This is his strength. This is what will make him a survivor, I tell myself. *If he can keep it up.* He must keep singing his own song, the foot therapy lady had said.

Then there's one of those rare and sudden moments of truth, when he tells you how worried he is. How frantic he is about the future. How frightened he is that he may not in the end be cured and how awful it is to be a cripple.

And how devastated he is that his dream to be a pilot has been smashed to smithereens.

You realise then that in spite of his positive attitude, his determination to get well, his herculean efforts to strengthen his leg, his tenacity in struggling to get more A-levels – inside he is scared stiff, and that hardly a day or night goes by when, if only for a fleeting moment, he is not terrified of the future.

If you do not know the truth, as only I do, you could be fooled.

We were over the sea now, having just passed Barcelona. I saw Andrew's face in the clouds and consoled myself with the knowledge that to confide in me this trickle of doubts and fears was to hasten his recovery. If he had to bottle them up they would surge into a torrential deluge of uncertainty. Only by telling me about them could they be diluted in the far stronger flow of his positive determination to overcome them.

I could not stay with him forever, but he still needed me. My presence was necessary, if only for this vital outlet. For those few occasions when he could tell me how he really felt.

Who else could he tell?

I felt the plane losing height and was jolted out of my thoughts.

Angry white horses pranced on the sea around Menorca's rocky coast. Dry stone walls and clusters of white villas gleamed in the sun, and a few minutes later, buffeted by a typical north easterly wind – the Tramontana – we touched down.

My old friends Christopher and Barbara were there to meet me, and greeting them was the catalyst for the unleashing of my tears. My outburst took me by surprise, and no matter how I tried I could not stop. Before driving me home they gave me tea and sandwiches at their flat, where at last I poured out the events of the past seven months.

- 0 -

I collected fifty and one hundred peseta pieces and phoned Andrew every day. And of course he was coping. So well, it seemed, that clearly I had worried for nothing.

From our house on the hill at S'Albufera d'Es Grau, the views are spectacular. To the north the lake, glinting like a giant sapphire in the sun. To the east the sea and the fragrant pine forest. And all around me the hills rolling like miniature Himalayas into the pale blue distance.

During the day I painted water-colours of the scenes I loved best, and at night friends took me out for dinner.

And in between I cried.

I don't know whether it was for Andrew or for myself – probably for us both and for the whole goddam terrible thing that had happened.

- 0 -

I always said that whenever I needed her most Jo would be there. Unbelievably she and Philip arrived in Menorca a week before I flew back to Manchester. Philip's calm, unruffled presence was soothing, while Jo's effervescence lifted me a little way out of my well of sadness.

I was longing to tell Jo about the dream.

I had wanted to tell her long ago but felt too ashamed. I had also wanted to tell Dr Jelliffe but had let the right moment slip by. I had told no one. Not even Colin. If only I could tell Jo now I knew she would help me to do something about it, especially here in leisurely Menorca,

200

where we had so much more time to talk.

I started going through the events of the dream in my mind, rehearsing them as it were for Jo. For some time now the ending had taken a new twist, leaving me with the agonising doubt that I would not succeed in plucking him back from that final exit. Suddenly I was questioning the facts of the dream, as though I had at last agreed to meet them face to face.

Alas. Facing them did not diminish the horror. Except that now it seemed there was room for these images to linger in my mind and I was able to allow them in without recoiling in terror and abomination. A sort of acceptance of my guilt, I suppose. (But why did I feel such guilt?)

I cried more after that, but I still didn't tell Jo.

- 0 -

At the end of the two weeks, I stopped crying. I was going back to Manchester and in the real world mothers didn't go around crying. I had to be strong and cheerful. Just as everyone knew I always would be.

I thought of what Jo had said, way back in March.

You will cope without ever wavering, with great strength and fortitude. But at the end you will probably have a nervous breakdown.

So was this it? A nervous breakdown? I had never thought her words could apply to me. I didn't know what nervous breakdowns were but whatever this was I think it did me a whole lot of good.

Not only did it alleviate the tension and grief for the suffering Andrew was enduring, and the separation that had been forced upon Colin and me, but my sense of outrage seemed to have melted away with my tears. My father once told me after he'd been treating a patient with what he called a nervous breakdown, that I would never suffer with such an affliction. Not his level-headed little daughter! Well, now I had – if that was what it was. But perhaps he had been certain that in our safe, well regulated life there would never be anything ghastly enough to cause me to break down.

I went back to Manchester revitalised. Before this 'breakdown', if anyone spoke to me about Andrew I would become emotional, defensive, unable to speak without a tremor in my lip. Now I felt I could face anyone and anything.

201

Well-armed, as it were, for the future slings and arrows of outrageous fortune.

- 0 -

"You didn't do all this on your own, did you, Andrew?"

"There's nobody else here but me," he said, grinning as he heaped my plate with slices of roast chicken and a colourful array of succulent vegetables which he had placed on the table even before I had unpacked my suitcase.

So, Peter had been right.

I also noticed how the muscles of his leg were growing and strengthening. Although it would never look like a normal leg, it no longer resembled a withered stick. I wanted to witness for myself how the physios at Withington Hospital were bringing about this transformation, so the following day I tagged along to see the splendid new rehabilitation wing, and Andrew in action.

I sat at the edge of the hydro-pool, surprised when all the other patients were cleared out before Andrew got in. I soon found out why. Moving through the water like a dolphin he looked as though he was in training for the Olympics. By the time he was finished the water level had dropped by several inches and I was soaking wet!

Each week he could bend the knee more and lift the leg higher, but by early November the physios had reached a deadlock; no matter how hard Andrew tried he could only lift his leg if it was first bent at an angle of thirty degrees. Nor could he bend the knee any more than forty-five degrees. Both these short-falls caused him to limp badly, and the prospects did not look good.

- 0 -

I sat at the dining-room table trying to put the finishing touches to the still-life water colour for tomorrow's Painting for Pleasure Class at the Adult Learning Centre in Withington I had recently joined. As I painted, I listened to the slow, deep notes of the cello that filled every room in the flat with a sound that seemed to come not so much from the instrument as from Andrew's very soul, reverberating through my body with a richness of tone that tore at my heart strings in the same way that a beautiful dancer made me gasp for breath.

202

Suddenly there was a false note and the music ended abruptly. A moment later there was a deep twang as though the instrument had fallen to the ground.

I knocked softly at the door of his room and entered.

"Why don't you do your Law homework instead, Andrew. You've been playing that tune for over an hour now. Maybe if you give it a break it'll –"

"Leave me alone, Mum. I don't want to do homework. It's so boring. Anyway, I'm playing my cello."

As he spoke he knelt down on his good knee and carefully picked up the cello from the floor. Whether he had thrown it down or it had fallen I do not know, but as his fingers touched the soft glowing wood they seemed to caress the instrument like a mother comforting her child.

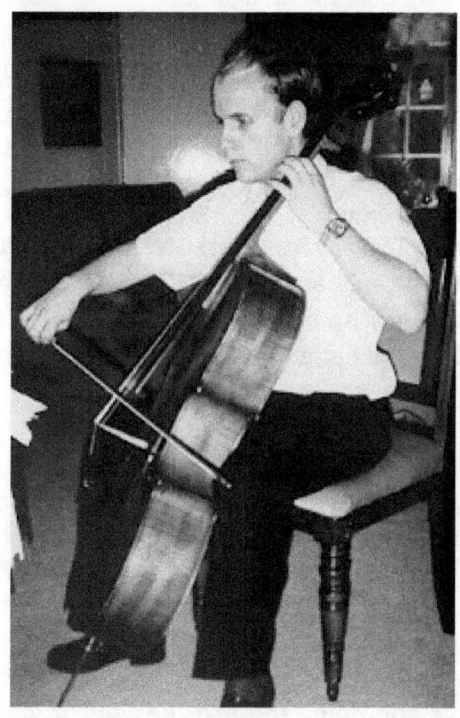

His music drives away the pain

- 0 -

Although situated in the shadow of Manchester's legal heart-land, I'd had a hunch for some time now that St John's College was not providing the necessary inspiration for Andrew to throw himself wholeheartedly into his A-level Law studies. Nevertheless I was only too pleased to see him go there every day. But winter was drawing in. Golden leaves were falling and piling up slippery on pavements, and lights were being switched on before four o'clock in the afternoons. Travelling was not easy for someone still not very steady on his feet.

One bleak, cold, grey morning, with the wind whistling through the bare branches and the rain hissing down, I stood at the window as I did every morning, and from the cosy warmth of the bedroom I watched Andrew limp across the road to the bus stop.

He could not run.

He would never be able to run again.

He just missed the bus.

With my index finger I cleared a small round patch in the misted up window. I saw his head sag into his turned-up raincoat collar. I saw his shoulders hunch as he waited for the next over-full bus.

And when it came I saw him struggle up the steps.

That night I phoned Colin.

Colin's philosophy has always been: Give them the flowers now!

"Buy him a car," he said at once. "He's not supposed to walk more than a few yards anyway, so buy him a car."

I blew Colin a kiss and hung up. I called Andrew away from his cello. I smiled at him.

"Do you think you could drive, Andrew?"

He frowned, then his eyes lit up and widened.

"You bet," he said breathlessly.

The next day we bought a pale blue Ford Fiesta. This would be his first opportunity to drive a car since getting both his Zambian and his English driving licences way back in January, only weeks before the trouble with his leg had become serious. If he hadn't succeeded then, there would have been little chance now of going through the rigours of learning to drive and doing the test. Besides, it was right now that he needed to drive.

We ordered a special accelerator to be fitted, but before we had even left the show-room Andrew decided to cancel it.

"The extra stretching movement to get my foot to the pedal might

204

actually do me good," he said.

I think too, that he didn't want any contraptions which would in any way label him 'disabled'.

That night Andrew put his arms around me. It was a long time since he'd looked so happy and excited. "A car of my own, Mum! I can't believe it!"

"Just you drive carefully," I said, biting my lip.

"Oh boy! No more missing the bus. No more getting on and off with crutches and a knee that won't bend properly. No more getting cold and wet ..."

"And no more excess walking which Mr Sweetnam has forbidden you to do," I said sternly.

It was not the whole answer. Parking in the centre of Manchester was difficult. And it may have been all the walking he had to do from distant car parks to the college that created yet another new problem.

Chapter Twenty-one

November 1984 – February 1985

I heard him scream.

My blood ran cold. It was the same nightmarish scream I used to hear before the operation, when Annabel was sawing off his leg.

I rushed to his room. Knelt by his bed. Held his hand. I did not need to ask what had happened.

I knew.

It was the middle of the night. His next check-up was tomorrow. Also, although Jo had often explained the difference between his treatment and Paul Grayson's, it was difficult for Andrew to forget that Paul had developed a secondary tumour in his lung one year after his operation.

And he knew that this was nearly always fatal.

- 0 -

In the Fracture Clinic waiting room Andrew sat staring at the wall, waiting to see Mr Sweetnam and Dr Jelliffe at their combined osteosarcoma clinic. We had left Manchester before dawn to travel up to London, and Andrew looked tired and pale. He spoke a few hushed words to a young girl he had first met on the ward, but otherwise there was absolute silence.

When he went to X-ray I sat watching the other bald teenagers, perched in a row on wooden benches like birds lashed by a winter's storm with nowhere else to go. I saw their sad eyes, their hunched shoulders, their thin concave chests. I looked from one solemn haggard pinched anxious face to another, wondering which of them would live to be one of the eighty-five percent survivors, and which would fall into the fifteen percent group that would die.

I wished I could comfort them all. I wished I could say to them all, *You're going to live! You can live. You all have a chance but you must*

206

be positive. You must be determined. You must never give up ...

Just then Jo arrived and snapped me out of it. As usual she always arrived when she was most needed, knowing instinctively just when those moments were. She knew too, that if Andrew got bad news he would need me to hold his hand, but he would need her to re-assure him medically.

Dressed only in a short, white, much washed cotton hospital garment, Andrew returned from X-ray. He sat down between us in the narrow corridor and stared at the wall. His face was sombre and unresponsive, just like all the others. He knew, as we all knew now, that if the chest X-ray was clear it meant there was no spread of the cancer.

And – vice versa.

One by one the other patients were swallowed up into the consulting room. The exit was through another door at the side, so I never found out if their anxiety had been quelled or not.

At last it was Andrew's turn. Mr Sweetnam greeted us cheerfully, his lean face alert, his dark brown eyes sparkling over the top of his glasses. Dr Jelliffe smiled warmly. The senior registrar was there too, and being a teaching hospital the room was full of students, gathered in a semi-circle around these two brilliant maestros.

Andrew clambered on to the narrow examination table. Mr Sweetnam was pleased with the general progress, but when Andrew tried the straight-leg lift he seemed perturbed to see the thirty degree lag which the physios in Manchester were trying so hard to eradicate. He then asked Andrew to walk across the room.

"Will he lose that limp soon?" I tried to sound as casual as possible.

Mr Sweetnam stroked his chin. "I doubt it. You see, you need a strong thigh muscle to lift the leg up straight, as we do when we walk. With any impairment or weakening of that muscle it is only possible to lift the leg by first bending the knee. Andrew has a plastic sling around his knee to hold the tendons, and because the sling is by necessity slightly too long he can only lift his leg with this thirty degree bend. In other words, the lag."

I narrowed my eyes. "But surely that will improve?"

"It may improve slightly," he said gently. "But I'm afraid he will probably always limp."

For me this was bad news, though everyone else present seemed to attach little importance to it. Even Andrew looked unconcerned, so

207

great was his relief that the chest X-ray, displayed prominently in the middle of the room, was pronounced clear.

Mr Sweetnam finished off his notes and asked Andrew to come back in three months' time.

A little later on I bumped into Dr Jelliffe in the hospital entrance hall.

"I'm very pleased with Andrew." He smiled his warm smile. "He's doing very well indeed. Mr Sweetnam seemed a little pessimistic about the limp but I think that with Andrew's youth and vitality and a lot of hard work, he should overcome it."

His words were like a gift from the gods. Andrew's eyes lit up when I told him, and a look of quiet determination settled on his face. I wonder if Dr Jelliffe knew how much that chance remark would boost Andrew's morale. He had not said much during the consultation, but now he had given Andrew all the incentive he needed.

"Yes!" Andrew said, with fire in his eyes. "I *will* get rid of this horrid limp."

- 0 -

Afterwards, while Andrew rushed off to greet old friends among the staff, Jo and I sat in the little tea-room where we always met, on the corner of Cleveland Street, adjacent to the hospital, savouring the good news.

I sipped my tea and gazed through the plate glass window at the never ending stream of traffic splashing through the puddles.

I smiled at Jo. "It's always such a relief when it's over, isn't it. And there's been no spread of the cancer," I added unnecessarily – unconsciously needing to reinforce in my own mind the positive result.

"It's natural to be on tenterhooks," she said, (and I knew there would be a proviso), "but you must never allow yourself to believe that they will give you bad news."

"I know." I nodded, thinking for the millionth time since Jo had first counselled me, how lucky I was to have her as a friend. "I always try to make sure Andrew knows this too, but I wish there was more of a cut-and-dried result of a check-up. They never say, Well, Andrew, you're absolutely fit and fine. They just nod their heads and say things are going well, report it all on their voice recorders and tell you to come back in two or three months' time."

208

"Nothing is cut and dried at this stage," Jo said, refilling my cup. "They can't tell you any more than they do. One day they'll extend that period to six months. Then it'll be one year. And before you know where you are he will have reached the five year mark."

"And what then?"

"Then you'll know he's cured."

- 0 -

Colin and I were a happily married couple but we were leading entirely separate lives. Though I missed him terribly the thought never entered my head that I should be with him in Lusaka. This was my life now. We all knew I had to be with Andrew.

Colin had some good friends in Lusaka, especially his two faithful golfing mates, Brian and Alan. They made life bearable for him, though I hate to think how many pints of beer the three of them sank on a Saturday night at the Golf Club.

Meanwhile, just as I had in London, I made the most of the music and art Manchester had to offer, and at the twice weekly 'Painting for Pleasure' class I attended I discovered to my delight that with perseverance anyone can paint!

All this helped to fill the gap. Neither of us knew how long our separation would last. We lived from day to day, an unnatural existence I did not dare to question. But we needed each other and I was becoming aware that the longer we stayed apart the more likelihood there was of our relationship changing.

- 0 -

During that first week at St John's College, when Andrew had come home one afternoon with a smile on his face and told me about his fellow student Julie, I was happy for him.

"Mum," he said, "I've met a really super girl."

"Oh!" I'd replied with an initial pang of fear, wanting to shield him, remembering the unknown girl who had fled from him on his way home from the pub. "That's nice. What's she like?"

"She's lovely, Mum. And she has fantastic eyes."

I looked at his own sunken eyes. I looked at his bald head. I looked at him from the point of view of this lovely girl with the fantastic eyes who couldn't possibly be attracted to him and who would surely reject him.

He had seemed to read my mind.

"Don't worry, Mum", he said. "I'm not going to fall in love with her."

The lovely Julie was in his Law class. One day he offered her a lift home and discovered she lived only a few minutes from our flat. Soon he was driving her to college in the mornings, and in the afternoons he brought her home to our flat for tea. She seemed fond of Andrew in a very shy and quiet way, and I felt myself warming to her.

"There's nothing in it, Mum. She has a boy-friend she's had for years. We're just good friends."

He played it 'cool', content to take a back seat, enjoying her company whenever he could. In his spare time he was fortunately occupied with his rifle shooting and his physiotherapy, but I think he was biding his time.

- 0 -

I saw little evidence of any concentrated work being done for the A-level Law course. It was a blessing that Peter and Andrea, both lawyers, could help him out with the odd problem because he had not yet regained the capacity for long hours of study. Besides, what would there be at the end of it? His life-long ambition had always been to be a pilot. Now he never mentioned it. Now there was nothing. Now it was a hopeless forgotten dream.

Or so I thought.

It amazed me that he continued to get out of bed morning after morning to sit through lectures which did not inspire him. Now and again, when I woke him at seven-thirty with his orange juice, he would jokingly say, "Mum, I don't want to go to school!" and snuggle down into the duvet. But five minutes later he'd be limping to the bathroom.

Then one day in late November he came home with a twinkle in his eye.

"Mum ... I'm in love!"

"Isn't she still seeing the other boy-friend?" I asked, immediately on my guard.

He gave me a sideways glance. "Yeah. But don't worry. That won't be for long."

210

Once again I tried to see him through the lovely Julie's cornflower blue eyes. Yes, he was beginning to put on weight, and yes, he was losing the wizened old-man look, but he still limped, and his new hair, instead of being straight and blond and shiny, was curly, mousy and dull.

One night we decided to measure it.

"One centimetre!"

I recorded this growth in my notebook, omitting to add that he looked like a punk rocker. When it was an inch and a half long it stuck out all over his head and I thought how very trendy he looked.

- 0 -

Andrew enjoyed more than anything the Monday and Wednesday nights when Uncle Stan took him to Altrincham Rifle club. I went with them once to see for myself how well he shot. Inside the range, with ear muffs on, I brimmed over with pride at his scores of ninety-six and ninety-seven.

He was still using Stan's rifle but longed to have his own and couldn't wait to get his licence.

One afternoon the door-bell rang. I found a friendly policeman and a policewoman on the doorstep, come at last to see Andrew about his application for a fire-arm licence; to assess his character and his suitability to own a dangerous weapon. The policewoman's gaze kept switching from the big framed photograph on top of the writing bureau, with the laughing blue eyes and shiny golden hair, to this sad-eyed young man with dull stubbly hair.

After several weeks the licence was at last ready. They brought it round personally to the flat, and minutes later Andrew drove into Manchester to buy his rifle.

What excitement when at his first big competition in Blackpool he won a silver cup. He was doing something he really enjoyed and his success pepped up his morale like a tonic. He is singing his own song, I thought, and smiled in wonder at the miracle of it all.

"He will be one of Dr Jelliffe's eighty-five percent group," I said aloud. "He will survive."

- 0 -

"No wonder you can't close your suitcase, Mum," Andrew said, hauling everything out in order to repack it for me. "Look at all this! Cheese. Chocolates. Christmas crackers!"

"Well, they're impossible to buy in Zambia. They haven't enough foreign exchange to import necessities, let alone luxuries."

At the last minute we even managed to squeeze in a packet of cherries, and when I was finally ready, Andrew took me to the airport.

He'd been thrilled when we planned to have a family Christmas in Zambia. He hadn't been back since early January and was longing to go home. He had a seat booked for three weeks later when the college term ended. I had worried about leaving so soon, but Peter and Andrea weren't far away, and Julie and he were often together now so he wouldn't be alone.

- 0 -

Lusaka was like a foreign country. Everything looked so different. I hadn't been home for ten months and I felt awkward and out of phase. Now that I was here I wasn't even sure I wanted to be here, and Colin and I had to learn to be together again.

For the first few days I was afraid our enforced separation might have damaged our relationship, made us too independent of one another. I had become used to living on my own and was quite self-sufficient. Now and then when we'd been apart I would suddenly realise that for a few days I hadn't even thought about Colin, because I was 'doing my own thing.'

In the end it had the opposite effect. The separation brought us closer together. Made us realise how much we meant to each other. The shared grief and worry about Andrew helped strengthen the bond between us. We didn't need to talk about it but it was there, binding us together.

But we also had violent arguments, very often about nothing at all, because of the tension we were both still living under.

Once I got used to it again it was good to be back in our lovely house in Kabulonga. In our quiet leafy street, hidden behind our glass-topped eight foot high wall with our lush green lawn, our black-faced yellow weaver birds busily weaving their hanging nests, our kidney shaped pool and our umbrella of brilliant flamboyant trees; I felt I was truly back in paradise.

212

Three weeks later we met Andrew at the airport. The sun had just burst into the sky and there was a faint mist rising from the dusty roads. There had been no rain since April and it was already too hot to breathe. Just as we arrived the big jet taxied in. A 'lollipop special' full of school children coming home for Christmas.

We raced up to the viewing balcony to catch a glimpse of him as he stepped off the plane, just as we had always done, three times a year ever since he first went to boarding school in Rhodesia at the age of six.

Only this time it was different.

Staring silently across the shimmering tarmac we watched the passengers spill down the steps.

Andrew was the last one to appear.

It was Andrew all right, but oh how different from the Andrew we had always seen leaping down the steps, first off the plane. This Andrew was thin, bent and slow. This Andrew walked with a limp.

When he saw us he waved his sticks, then drew himself up straight and walked proudly across the tarmac into the terminal building.

We stood behind the big glass doors, waiting, and suddenly he was wheeling his trolley towards us.

"At least he hasn't lost his knack of getting through Customs and Immigration faster than anyone else," Colin said, shaking his head in amazement.

"In spite of his wonky leg."

I hugged him till my eyes filled with tears. I had missed him so much.

Once outside the building he stopped. He leaned on his sticks and took a long, deep breath.

"I'm home!" he said. "I'm home ... I never thought I would be." There was a tremor in his voice.

When we arrived at the house he walked round and round the garden, looking at the trees and the flowers, talking and joking with Sarah, his old nanny, and Adam the cook, and hugging Fifi who squirmed and wriggled and wagged her tail with delight.

Christmas came and went, and all too soon it was time to go back for the new term at St John's.

At the airport I hid behind my sunglasses until the plane was out of sight.

I flew back to England in time for Andrew's next check-up at The Middlesex. Instead of the usual combined clinic, he would be seeing Dr Jelliffe on Thursday afternoon and Mr Sweetnam on Friday. He had the usual nightmare the night before, but as our Inter-City train sped southwards to London he seemed quite calm, and there was nothing untoward that could have warned us of the drama to come.

- 0 -

Like Mr Sweetnam, Dr Jelliffe treats each patient as an individual. He always has time to listen and is delighted with Andrew's progress and impressed that he is studying so soon for his A-levels.

"Go and have your X-rays now, Andrew. Mr Sweetnam will examine them when he sees you tomorrow morning. I'll see you again in three months' time."

But instead of the usual X-ray room next to the orthopaedic clinic, today we must go to the general X-ray department, with its long queue of diverse patients.

"I can't stand this waiting, Mum. It's driving me mad. Do we have to stay?"

At last the nurse calls him in.

I wait in my usual numb state. I read tattered copies of *Woman's Own* and *The Illustrated London News*. I try not to look at my watch or allow my thoughts to stray into forbidden land.

When Andrew finally appears his face is filled with indignation.

"They won't let me see the X-rays!"

Normally this is not a problem as they are displayed prominently in the middle of Mr Sweetnam's room for everyone to see, minutes after they are taken.

"Calm down, Andrew."

He sits next to me. "They're sending the plates directly to Mr Sweetnam's clinic. I have to wait until tomorrow to see them." He bounces up again. "No. I can't wait that long. I'm going to look at them now. Before they send them off."

In a few minutes he is back with a look of such horror on his face that I think he is going to faint.

He flops into the chair next to me.

"I've had it, Mum," he says quietly.

"What do you mean?"

"There's a big spot on my chest X-ray."

My stomach turns. "You're imagining it, Andrew."

"I'm not. I've seen it. I must go back to Dr Jelliffe and find out what's happening. I'm not leaving the hospital until I know."

He had arranged to meet Nicola, but now only one thing matters.

We walk down the long, wide, crowded corridor to the other side of the hospital. The resounding clunk of his sticks echoes on the polished floor like stones being thrown down a cliff into a deserted valley. I hear no other sounds. See no other people. For me only Andrew exists.

I press the call-bell for the lift. We stand in silence. I steal a glance at his taut, drawn features. What about the chemotherapy? I wonder indignantly. It had nearly killed him but it was also supposed to have killed any stray cancer cells that might have spread to his lungs.

Had all that been for nothing?

I think of the one and three-quarter treatments he never had. Suppose ... suppose he – Oh no!

I take a deep breath. The fifteen percent non-survival rate has been hanging over our heads for so many months now. It was never really far away, was it? After all, Dr Jelliffe said right at the beginning that he only had an eighty-five percent chance of survival ...

Does this mean he is now one of the doomed fifteen percent?

My negative thoughts are interrupted by the clanging arrival of the lift. Dr Jelliffe's secretary, who protects him so infuriatingly from over-anxious pestering mothers of patients, says if she can find him he will see us in the little consulting room where nearly a year ago he told us Andrew's leg might after all have to be amputated. So, he was wrong then, wasn't he? He could be wrong again. He's not infallible, even though he is the best.

We sit in the empty waiting room. My morbid thoughts sear into every crevice of my mind like lava flowing from a volcano. Unstoppable. Relentless. All-enveloping.

No! I tell myself. *Stop it. Andrew knows me too well. I must exude a confident exterior or he will begin to panic.*

We wait. Five o'clock comes and goes. Five-thirty. Six. Still no Dr Jelliffe. Then his secretary comes in. She has located him at another hospital. He is unable to come now, but is sending one of his housemen who is familiar with the case.

215

Half an hour later the houseman arrives. She is very understanding and kind. She promises to try to get the X-rays but if this is impossible Andrew will have to wait until he sees Mr Sweetnam tomorrow morning.

"No!" Andrew says. "I must know now! I'm not leaving until I know."

He is being a damned nuisance but he is facing square-on the possibility of a spread of the cancer, knowing it could be fatal. He does not want to run away from the truth. He wants to know whether he is going to live or die.

My heart goes out to him and I love him more now than it has ever seemed possible to do. I gaze at his face. Although his aggression and his fierce determination are tinged with fear there is also a look of intrepid defiance that almost frightens me.

"Not tomorrow morning," he says again. "*Now!*"

The doctor can see he means what he says. She hurries away in search of the X-rays. As I pick up my notebook, Nicola arrives.

She sits close to Andrew.

"I'm sure I saw mets on the X-ray," he whispers. "I'm not going to have chemo again. I can't –"

"Don't be silly, Andrew." She holds his hand. Says the only thing she can say. "There won't be anything there, I bet you. And even if it has metastasised, you'll be okay."

The three of us do our best to keep up a light-hearted conversation. Every now and then Andrew and Nicola whisper. At last, at seven o'clock, we hear the lift approaching. We sit rock still.

The metal door jangles open.

The high heels tap-tap across the lobby, then up the steps to the waiting room.

She appears in the doorway.

I hold my breath.

My head swims.

Will this be it?

She smiles at Andrew. His jaw is like a vice, his knuckles like polished white pebbles.

"The X-rays are perfectly clear, Andrew. Everything is fine."

I murmur thank you, but Andrew's face says it all.

- 0 -

I stood watching Andrew go off arm-in arm with attractive, vivacious, warm-hearted, compassionate Nicola, smiling happily with his old friend as they walked away from the hospital towards a restaurant in Henrietta Street where she had booked a table. As they disappeared into the night and I was left standing alone on the edge of the curb, I suddenly realised how pathetic I must look.

He's okay, isn't he? Well, for God's sake, woman. Be happy. Smile!

I was still smiling as I walked on to the dusty platform at Goodge Street tube station. In front of me was a huge advertisement pasted onto the curved wall of the tunnel, inviting everyone to give generously to the Cancer Research Fund. Then there was a sudden roar, and a rush of hot air that blew my long brown hair across my eyes as the train for Highgate snaked to a hissing stop.

I shuffled on and found a seat. Opposite me the distorted reflection of my face in the window smiled. It smiled crookedly all the way to Highgate. I couldn't wait to tell Jenny the wonderful news.

- 0 -

Next morning Andrew and I arrived at the clinic waiting room just before nine-thirty, and Jo breezed in a few minutes later.

As we entered Mr Sweetnam's room my eyes were drawn to the illuminated X-ray which almost jumped out of its frame to attract my attention.

I could see no ominous looking spot, though with its mass of squiggles I could understand how easily Andrew had imagined the worst. I smiled but at the same time I felt a tremble shudder through my body. For Andrew – whatever it was he saw yesterday – it had been real.

Mr Sweetnam was also pleased with Andrew's progress and commented on the limp which he could see was not as pronounced as in November. We left with an appointment card for the end of April. This meant he would have all of May and June ahead of him, free of worry and tension so that he could study with a clear and untroubled mind for July's A-level exams.

Or so I imagined.

217

Chapter Twenty-two

February – June 1985

"Colin was right when he said Andrew behaves like an oil sheik's son," Peter said as he carved the Sunday joint. "You do too much for him, Mum. You're too soft with him."

"And why not?" I said, always on the defensive where Andrew was concerned. "After what he's been through he deserves it. He's still under a lot of stress, what with his check-ups every two or three months. Colin is probably jealous of his brother because I never spoilt him. Or you," I added, giving him a playful punch on the arm.

Peter shook his head. "You're creating a life-style for Andrew which won't prepare him for the harsh realities of life. If you don't make him study hard now and get good grades and go on to university, he'll never amount to anything. He should be working at it now, instead of going out gallivanting."

Andrew was out with Julie, and Peter and Andrea had invited me for lunch.

"Can't you see he's just being lazy, Mum? He's not trying. He has no ambition to succeed in these exams."

I thought about this. "The problem is he's just not serious about Law. More A-levels, yes, but all he ever wanted to do was fly. There's no specific goal to aim for now. In his present state he can't see himself slogging away at a Law degree. He wants to get on with life. He can't afford to waste all that time."

Peter looked unconvinced. "How do you know all this? Has he told you?"

"He doesn't need to. I know. I also know the last thing he needs now is stress. Cancer cells thrive on stress."

Peter raised his eyebrows. "I thought you said he had no cancer cells left."

"I don't think he has, but you can't afford to take the slightest chance. I don't want anyone forcing him to 'get on with it'. Later, yes.

218

If he survives." The words were out before I could stop myself. Words I always tried so hard not to think about. I bit my lip to steady it and breathed in deeply. "Dr Jelliffe told me the first two years were when he would be the most vulnerable. After that the chances of it spreading will rapidly decrease with each six months, until at the five year mark he should be free. If there's anything under the sun I can do to lessen that vulnerability then I'm jolly well going to do it."

"And that includes spoiling?"

"If it prevents stress, yes,"

Peter's tone softened. "It was a cruel twist of fate for this happen in his final school year, but that doesn't mean he can sit back now. He has to make up for lost time."

I smiled. Clearly Peter and I were never going to agree on this.

"Anyway, I think it's high time you left him to get on with things himself. He's getting stronger and fitter by the week. You should go back to Zambia, Mum." He had put into words what I'd been thinking for some time now.

"I know. Though I really want to be around during the exams. To see that he eats properly and gets there on time. Remember how Colin missed a vital exam by going a day late?"

"I remember." He pursed his lips. "But that will be leaving it too long."

"Oh, if only my home wasn't five thousand miles away I could come and go as I'm needed." I sighed deeply. "Do you think he'll be courageous enough to go through with the exams, knowing he hasn't really worked as hard as he needed to?"

"You'll just have to hope that he will. But if you stay you'll be robbing him of the freedom he so badly needs to face the world again. Alone. As a man."

Peter was right.

I made my plans, finally convincing myself that I had become superfluous. He had Peter and Andrea. He had Julie. He had college every day. He had Uncle Stan and the rifle club.

It was good that he had the shooting. The foot reflexology therapist in London had said he should sing his own song. Doing something well, that you enjoyed doing was part of this philosophy. You had to believe in yourself; you had to know where you were going; you had to follow this path knowing it was what you wanted in order to achieve your goals. And that it was *you* who had mapped it out.

The foot lady would be pleased. Andrew was not feeling sorry for himself. He was determined to get better. This was priority number one.

There was only one problem.

He still had no goal.

Or so I thought.

None of us ever spoke about the tragedy of the lost flying career, least of all Andrew. But he would have to do *something*. We discussed this, and before I left I persuaded him to start writing letters of application to banks. He was always honest in his letters, explaining quite frankly about his illness though stressing that he had now recovered.

At last he got an interview at a well-known bank in Manchester. In his best dark suit he set off, full of enthusiasm. He had all the qualifications required, and much more.

"How did it go?" I asked when he arrived home.

His eyes were sparkling. "It went really well. I reckon I'll get the job."

Jo and I chatted about this on the phone. She was against him applying for jobs at this early stage.

"He's not ready yet to be exposed to the cut-throat world of job hunting. Just look at him. He looks half-starved. He's as weak as a kitten and his hair ... well ... it doesn't do anything for him, does it?"

She was adamant. "It's not fair to offer himself in a highly competitive market against fit and well opponents. Rejections at this stage could cause him to lose confidence in himself."

"Jo, he doesn't see himself as anything but fit and well. He no longer has cancer! He has recovered! And he can't see that he looks anything but normal."

"I know," she said. "Anyway, Andrew will be wasted in a bank. He should be in the hotel industry. Where his personality will be so special that any hotel he works for will have guests queuing to get back in!"

Dear Jo. She had great expectations for Andrew's future. She was frequently his guide, his confidante, his mentor, and he always phoned her about a crisis or a success or a new development. Often his tenacity and determination were inspired by Jo, but she never took any nonsense from him and never ever gave him sympathy.

A week later a letter arrived in the early post. I took it in with the orange juice and stood by the bed while he ripped it open. It wasn't difficult to see at a glance that in those few lines there was no offer of a job. In disgust he screwed it up and threw it on the floor.

Right then I could have killed that bank manager.

Soon afterwards I read in a Sunday newspaper about a bank that sacked a young employee because he had not told them he'd had cancer, even though he had now recovered. The bank was quoted saying it was not their policy to employ people with illnesses likely to result in extended periods off work.

So were they all clairvoyants I wondered? Did they have crystal balls? Anybody could get ill. At any time. Anybody could have an accident. How could you discriminate against somebody just because they had once been ill?

With my blood boiling I realised this article explained a great deal about Andrew's rejections, which were now flowing in thick and fast.

Without the offer of a job, or even a vague promise, there continued to be little incentive to work for A-levels. He had tried every bank in the country, the civil Service and the Foreign Office. With the Air Force out of the question things were looking pretty bleak. And with not even a glimmer of hope he was doing less and less studying at home.

- 0 -

In the middle of March I unwillingly boarded a British Caledonian flight for Lusaka.

With a strange feeling of unrest in my mind.

- 0 -

Once more breathing in the clean, fresh, African air my spirits soared. It was so good to be home and oh so good to be with Colin again.

But my heart was cleft in two. One half wishing I was still with Andrew.

Sensing the conflict, Colin was patient. "He'll be fine," he said gently. "He's probably out with his friends right now, celebrating being on his own!"

It didn't help to know that my husband was almost certainly right.

I counted the days to the twenty-fifth of April, the day of Andrew's next check-up. I was relieved that Jo had offered to 'hold his hand', for

221

even the joy of being back in Zambia had not dispelled the strange feeling I'd been having lately that all was not well. To most people it must sound absurd that a nineteen-year-old could not go alone to the doctor, but these were not ordinary visits. There was always that fifteen percent possibility of being told the cancer had spread, or he must have another operation. Or both. He needed someone who loved him enough to share this agony with him.

At seven-thirty that evening we sat down on either side of the telephone. Colin poured us a beer. When the froth had settled we had a few quick gulps, then I dialled Jo's number in London.

Sometimes it was impossible to get through to the UK but yes, there was the connecting click and now it was ringing ...

"He's okay! Everything's okay!" were Jo's first words.

We slept well that night, and I bet Andrew did too.

- 0 -

Secrets were unheard of in our family.

Regular phone calls kept us in touch. Andrew said he was working as hard as he could, so how were we to know he had already discovered something which must have made it impossible for him to study at all?

From five thousand miles away it sounded as though he was coping more than adequately. I told myself I had worried for nothing, yet at other times I reproached myself for leaving him alone. I would lie awake planning to fly the very next day, then in the morning tell myself to stop being ridiculous and leave him to get on with it.

That is what one half of me said.

The other, inner, more discerning half kept saying that I should be with him.

I only knew later that the other, inner, more discerning half had been right all along.

But I did not go back. I had to conform. Peter had said mothers of nineteen-year-olds were not supposed to 'baby' their sons.

- 0 -

There was one small crisis the day before the exams started.

Sarah had just brought in my tray of tea when the phone rang. My

222

heart lurched when I heard his distraught voice.

"I feel terrible, Mum. My leg is painful. I can't keep anything down ..."

In the split second after I heard those words every detail of my ghastly dream flashed across my mind. You see, I said to myself, you *should* have stayed. Then I took a deep breath and pulled myself together.

Exam nerves, I thought. *Simple as that.* "You'll feel better tomorrow, Andrew," I said gently but as firmly as I could. "Sometimes being nervous makes you feel that way. It's quite natural but you'll get over it, my darling."

I took a large gulp of my hot steaming Rooibos tea, then I went on saying all the comforting things I could think of, trying to spark off the strength he needed to go through with it. Strength I knew he had but which had clearly vanished with this sudden glitch in his confidence.

I was used to these sudden bouts of depression and anxiety, which were so unlike the old, happy Andrew. But they were far fewer now, thank goodness, than when he first came out of hospital, when the fear that lurked beneath the surface had often erupted in an uncharacteristic display of emotion. But on this occasion he wisely telephoned and got it off his chest, then proceeded to snap out of it.

Further phone calls confirmed that his mysterious ailment had disappeared. He got up early the next day, drove into the city, parked outside St John's College now that he had a disabled badge, and wrote the first exam. A week later they were all over, and I breathed a sigh of relief.

- 0 -

When you are dealing with an illness like cancer you have to live from day to day, taking each one as it comes.

You have to be prepared for ups and downs.

223

Chapter Twenty-three

June 1985 – January 1986

As soon as the exams ended Andrew flew home to Lusaka. It would just be a short visit, he said, as he'd arranged to take five friends, including the lovely Julie, to Menorca in July, but he knew how very much we wanted to see him first.

Looking back, he must also have wanted to see us very much.

Shivering in the cool dry winter breeze that swept over Lusaka's deforested plains, we stood watching the passengers streaming down the steps from the aircraft, hurrying across the tarmac to be first in line to get through the tedious formalities demanded of passengers arriving in Zambia.

"There he is!" said Colin, when Andrew was almost in the terminal building. I would have missed him altogether because I'd been looking for a skinny lad with short mousy hair and a limp. This one had long blond hair, his head was held high and there was almost no trace of a limp.

We grinned at each other, then turned and ran downstairs.

- 0 -

Andrew was thrilled that we'd planned to spend the weekend at Kariba, that huge man-made lake between Zimbabwe and Zambia that is more like a sea than a lake. He was even more thrilled that my sister Muriel, husband John and their youngest daughter Bridget were driving up from Harare to join us at the Lake View Hotel on the Zimbabwe side of the lake.

We planned to leave on Friday morning, but just before we left we were suddenly catapulted to the brink of an abyss that threatened to suck the three of us into its treacherous depths.

- 0 -

It is six in the morning. The weaver birds are starting to sing so I tiptoe to the kitchen to make a pot of tea. As I pass Andrew's bedroom he explodes through the door, almost knocking me off my feet.

He stares at me with terrified eyes.

I slam down the tray, spilling the milk. I take his hands in mine. "What on earth —"

"I've had it, Mum." The words erupt from his mouth in a voice that is not his own.

"What?"

"There's a lump," he says, and crumples into my arms.

I hold him tight. I whisper, "Where?"

"At the top of my leg."

I breathe slowly. I must calm him down. I must make him feel safe. I am falling off the edge of a cliff but I don't want him to fall off too.

"It'll be all right, darling," I say, and lead him to our bedroom.

There is a quality of unreality that removes me from reality and levitates me to the ceiling. I look down as though I am watching a scene from a play. I do this often. My way of calming myself down in the face of a catastrophe.

Andrew sits on the edge of the bed, next to his father. His mother sits on the other side. The father looks at the mother. Frowns. The mother shakes her head. The light is shining through the big yellow flowers on the curtains and she walks over stiffly and opens them to let in the sun, as though this will somehow diffuse the horror and the fear.

"What is it, son?" the father says.

"A lump, Dad. At the top of my leg." He has stopped shaking.

"Let me see it."

Sure enough, there it is. At the top of the misshapen leg. About the size of a large marble.

"Have you only just discovered it?" the father asks.

"No."

"When?"

"Just after my last check-up at The Middlesex."

My brain whizzes round in circles. Jo had been with him that day. Everything had been fine. He'd been clear.

"But that was two months ago!" I say, from above.

Then I realise that for two months he has kept this knowledge to

225

himself.

For two months he must have had feelings of despair. For two months we had thought he was just fine, working for his A-levels, perfectly happy and normal.

Why did he keep it to himself?

I float down and put my arm around him. He is going through a crisis of emotion – a mixture of relief and agony. Relief because he no longer has to bear the burden of the knowledge of the lump all by himself. Agony because telling us has made it a fact. When it was a secret he could hide it away. Bury it. Pretend it did not exist.

Now it is real.

Now it must be confronted.

I look at his face. So young, yet so tormented. I look at Colin's face. It is grey with worry. He holds Andrew's hand tightly.

"What are you going to do, son?"

"Go and see Dr Jelliffe, Dad. As soon as possible"

"Good thinking," Colin says. "There's a flight tomorrow."

"No, Dad. Not yet."

Typical of the new Andrew, the thoughtful Andrew, the considering-other-people Andrew, his foremost thought is for us.

"First we'll go to Kariba, as you and Mum planned. I'm not going to mess up everyone's holiday."

- 0 -

Before we left I took Andrew to the company clinic to see our GP.

He examined the lump.

He did not look very happy. "It's probably just a reaction to something, causing an enlargement of a lymph gland ..."

I closed my eyes and breathed a sigh of relief.

"However ..."

He sucked in his breath.

"It might be malignant, so it must be looked at soon."

The yellow walls of the consulting room swayed towards me. I glanced at Andrew. Fear had transformed his face into a melting rubber mask and I could see that he too was teetering on the edge of a big black empty hole – a void that was sucking him into an unknown bottomless pit.

226

Beautiful Kariba Dam.

The largest man-made dam in the world. A gigantic concrete and steel wall spanning the mighty Zambezi River. Created in the 1950s to generate power for Central Africa, flooding hundreds of miles of land, causing thousands of people to be resettled away from their ancestral homes, and six thousand wild animals to be rescued and relocated in Operation Noah.

Now there were hundreds of miles of blue 'sea', with proper waves and purple mountains in the distance; with fish and birds and boats and the gentle lapping sounds of water. Like an oasis in the Sahara, an island in the Pacific, it was to us in landlocked Zambia a miracle: a tropical beach paradise.

After months in wintry dusty dry Lusaka it was an uplifting sight. Sipping our ice cold lagers on the wide veranda of the Lake View Hotel, with the whispering palm trees framing the seemingly endless expanse of 'sea', the euphoria induced by these delightful surroundings anaesthetised our troubled minds.

Andrew's cousin Bridget was seventeen. So like Andrew with her blonde hair and her blue eyes and her wide, heart-stopping smile that they could have been brother and sister. She was someone his own age with whom to share his present plight, and they spent the whole idyllic weekend together, swimming and fishing and talking. And sometimes laughing.

The three hour drive back to Lusaka boomeranged us back to reality. I was haunted by the fear of Andrew having to go through the appalling treatment which a positive diagnosis would set in motion.

He did not deserve this further blow.

The first thing he did after walking into the house back in Lusaka was to phone Philip and Jo Rodin in London. Thank goodness the temperamental Zambian phone was working. He explained the symptoms in detail and Philip told him it was unlikely this lump would be malignant. He gave two reasons.

"It just isn't typical of the pattern of osteosarcoma, Andrew. Secondly, enlarged lymph glands, which I'm almost certain this is, are two-a-penny, so at your age I don't think this is anything to worry about." He paused. "But at this distance I cannot possibly be absolutely certain. You must see Dr Jelliffe as soon as possible."

227

Andrew was a bit more relaxed after talking to Philip, but when he telephoned Dr Jelliffe, his over-zealous secretary refused to let Andrew speak to him, though she did promise to squeeze him into the already full appointment list for next Monday – the day he'd be in London on his way to Menorca.

Andrew was distraught. He needed the oncologist's re-assurance. It was quite unreasonable of her to treat him like this when she knew he was five thousand miles away.

I also tried to phone him, and so did Philip from London, but even he was unable to get past the secretary. I was seething.

Andrew left Zambia on Sunday night. We hugged him and he clung to us, too choked up to speak. His brave smile was the last thing I saw before he disappeared through the smudgy glass doors into the departure lounge. When we walked out to watch the plane disappear into the star-studded sky, tears filled my eyes.

"I should be going with him."

Colin put his arm around my shoulders. "Stop worrying," he said, and I consoled myself that Julie would be at Heathrow at six-thirty tomorrow morning to escort him to the hospital, and hold his hand.

We had a bad twenty-four hours waiting for news. That night the dream came back in Technicolor and I woke up bathed in sweat and clutching Colin. The next day Colin went to work and I wandered aimlessly around the house and garden with Fifi in my arms, hugging her and talking to her, and she, clever little Poodle, licking my face as though that would calm my fears. I was terrified to use the phone in case Andrew was trying to get through from London.

Fraught with worry Colin came home unprecedentedly early. If all was well Andrew should already be on his four-thirty flight to Menorca. If not ... well, we would soon find out.

We had arranged to phone Philip and Jo at seven. On the dot we dialled their number. Peep Peep Peep. Oh no! There were no free international lines.

A minute later we tried again.

Through the wide open windows the frogs croaked and the crickets chirped and the wind whistled through the flamboyant trees, rustling their feathery fronds.

Finally, at seven-thirty, we got through.

"He's fine!" Jo shouted through the crackles. "Dr Jelliffe thinks it's an enlarged lymph gland. He told Andrew to go ahead and have his

228

holiday, but to take it very, very easy and see him again as soon as he gets back."

"Thank you, Jo," I said, and collapsed in a heap into Colin's arms.

- 0 -

Two weeks later we flew to Manchester on the first leg of Colin's annual long leave, and the following week Andrew arrived back in Manchester from his holiday in Menorca. He looked fitter and happier than he had for more than a year and a half, but it was abundantly clear that Dr Jelliffe's instructions to 'take it very, very easy' had not been obeyed.

On Thursday we all went up to London for his check-up at the combined clinic. First Andrew went for X-rays then the three of us trooped into the consulting room together.

All eyes were on the illuminated frame.

Dr Jelliffe and Mr Sweetnam both thought the enlarged lymph gland could be the result of a slight movement of the metal prosthesis at the point where it fitted into the remaining tip of the tibia.

Andrew nodded. "Now and then I feel a sensation of rotation. It hurts like hell."

Dr Jelliffe said the lymph gland was probably reacting to this irritation, doing its job by acting as a barrier in trapping any microbes travelling up along the lymphatic system from the seat of the trouble. Mr Sweetnam looked sternly at Andrew over the top of his glasses. "You have a sub-standard leg, Andrew. You must treat it very gently, and with great respect."

"Yes, Sir," Andrew said guiltily.

I hoped this advice would really sink in this time, yet I had an uneasy feeling that something was not quite right with the reconstructed leg.

Next came the lung X-ray.

We held our breath.

Yes! It is clear!

So apart from the swollen gland, or what they thought was a swollen gland, they seemed quite sure that there was nothing to worry about.

So much so that Colin and I felt confident that we could now go and relax and enjoy our holiday in Menorca.

229

Colin let the sand trail through his fingers. It was a blisteringly hot August day on Son-Bou beach. He raised his glass and we drank to Peter and Andrea's first wedding anniversary – and to Andrew's health.

"What an improvement in just one year," Colin said, and I could still see the pale thin waif in the pale grey drooping suit, trying to enjoy the wedding, grasping his two sticks, his bald head held high and the white wisps of hair sticking up over the sad, dark eyes.

"An incredible difference," I said, plucking a juicy grape from the bunch as I recalled the moment he had rung the bell on his arrival back from his holiday a few weeks ago, when I'd rushed down to open the door, hardly believing the sight before my eyes – the happiest smile I had ever seen, the golden bronze face, eyes sky blue and sparkling, the sun-bleached hair, shiny and wavy and almost down to his shoulders ...

We lay back on the hot sand, our feet in the turquoise water, looking up at the cloudless sky and listening to the gentle swish of the waves – revelling in our happiness that he was alive.

Then a few days later came the fantastic news.

"I've passed my A-level Law!"

- 0 -

Colin flew to Lusaka and I went back to Manchester. Now that Andrew had left St John's College he had to decide what to do. I wanted to help if I could.

Getting a job was uppermost in his mind. He desperately wanted to be independent. He needed to prove to himself that he *could* get a job. He needed to prove his normality.

He was far too impatient to think in the long term, so, much to his father's disappointment, the idea of following in Peter's footsteps in the law profession was now out of the question. So was any other career that might delay his independence. He wanted to stand on his own two feet. He wanted to quench his thirst for living.

He wrote again to all the banks. He wrote to the building societies and the insurance companies. He scoured the *Manchester Evening News* small ads. The more letters he wrote the more rejections came in, or they ignored his applications altogether.

One night in disgust he swished the pile of letters off the table and they fluttered to the floor like the forlorn carriers of bad news that they were.

"I'm wasting my time, Mum," he said angrily. "I don't even want to work in a bank. I want to fly aeroplanes!"

I bit my lip. It had been his earliest ambition. Nothing else had sparked his interest. "Well, you know that's impossible now," I said firmly.

Just to make quite sure that no stone was left unturned we checked with several friends closely connected with the RAF. They all confirmed that Andrew would never be accepted for flying training, even though at seventeen he'd been offered the prestigious RAF flying scholarship.

"Okay," Andrew said sensibly. "No flying. That's pretty final. But what now?"

Then a new idea began to formulate in the back of his mind.

"What about a career in the airline industry? If I can't be a pilot, at least I could work closely with aircraft."

With eyes sparkling and cheeks glowing he reminded me of the idle chat he'd had with a friend of ours in Lusaka, the area manager of British Caledonian Airways in Zambia, during that brief tumultuous visit in June when the lump was revealed. Andrew had told him how impossible it was to get a job without any work experience, and Ray had very kindly said Andrew could work for a few months with the airline in Lusaka. To get something on his CV.

Unfortunately he could not take up the B Cal offer then because another check-up at The Middlesex was due. Besides, he really wanted to get a job on his own merit, one that nobody helped him to get. This was very important to him. It was part of the process of re-establishing himself as an individual. Part of 'singing his own song'.

Every night he combed the Employment Offered columns in the Manchester Evening News.

"*Anything* will do, Mum. *Anything* in the airline or travel industry."

- 0 -

I flew back to Lusaka and left Andrew with his job hunting, urging him to give up and come out to Zambia as soon as possible where he knew he could at least have some unpaid training with British Caledonian.

231

In the middle of October he went to London for the combined clinic. Jo was there to hold his hand if necessary, and when we phoned that night she told us everything was fine.

"They're still not unduly worried about the lump" she said, "although they are keeping an eye on it. Andrew was very confident this time."

This was good news. It was getting better all the time.

- 0 -

After weeks of fruitless job hunting Andrew gave up. "I can't get anything in the airline or travel industry without previous experience," he said. "So I've booked to come home on the eleventh. I'm really looking forward to working for B Cal."

Ten days before he flew, Colin and I were relaxing on the patio at the end of another sweltering day with our bare feet dangling in the pool and our ice cold lagers in our hands. Suddenly the telephone jangled into life.

We charged up the steps, guessing it might be Andrew.

"I've got a job! I've got a job!"

Colin thrust his fist high into the air. "Well done, son!"

I grabbed the phone. "Congratulations, darling ... Oh! What did you say? ... A temporary job? ... For one week only? With an insurance company ...?"

The modesty of the job and its brevity did not seem to have dampened Andrew's elation. "What's wrong, Mum? I'll work my week and I'll still come home on the eleventh."

We wished him luck and said goodbye, then burst out laughing. Partly in relief, partly in astonishment, but mostly because we were so happy for him.

"Well I'll be damned," Colin said. "He's done it in spite of everything. The stigma of the illness, his disability, the high unemployment rate, no experience ..."

I buried my head in Colin's shoulder.

- 0 -

From the moment Andrew started working for B Cal in Lusaka he loved every minute of it.

232

At the end of the first week he said, "That's it, Mum. I've made up my mind. I'm going to be an airline man."

He got up at six every morning and Colin dropped him off at the B Cal offices in Cairo Road, that wide bustling colossus of a street that is the hub of Lusaka. The days were long and busy and exciting, especially on Mondays and Thursdays when the flights arrived from London in the early morning and flew out again late the same night. On those days he worked a fourteen hour day at the airport, never complaining of his leg even though he was on his feet for hours on end. It was what he wanted to do and he was happy.

A Dutch friend whose children always travelled B Cal told us Andrew was very good at his job.

"He's so good," she said, "that he could talk anybody into flying B Cal even if they didn't want to go anywhere at all!"

- 0 -

At last he could add that magic word to his CV.

Experienced.

This in theory should open the door to further employment, but in the airline industry competition was fierce, so it wasn't easy for Andrew to leave Lusaka for the uncertainties of the big wide world.

Unfortunately he had no option. Another check-up at The Middlesex was due and he had to go.

In those seven happy weeks, nobody, least of all Andrew, had mentioned the lump.

233

Chapter Twenty-four

January – February 1986

A few days after he arrived back in Manchester Andrew got a job in a travel agency doing reservations and ticketing. He got it on the strength of the B Cal experience and Ray's glowing reference, but the pay was low and the prospects of advancement non-existent.

"It's okay," he said when I rang a week later. "It fills a gap but I want a real job, Mum. I want to work for a big airline."

But how would he get into an airline?

On B Cal Lusaka's recommendation he got an interview at their head office in London, and a few days later was thrilled when American Airlines also asked him for an interview.

Things were looking up.

- 0 -

I was born in Cape Town and for many years had been dreaming of going back to see my old friends and my beloved Table Mountain. Andrew was well, he had a job, albeit not the one he wanted, and it seemed at last I was free to realise my dream.

Cape Town was as magical as ever. As a treat I stayed at the Mount Nelson, the old colonial hotel with a reputation as old and colourful as that of Raffles in Singapore, the Norfolk in Nairobi and the Victoria Falls Hotel in Zimbabwe. The imposing pink buildings at the top of Government Avenue were hidden among the giant leafy oaks on the lower slopes of Table Mountain and I'd always thought how heavenly it would be to stay there.

I was not disappointed.

I visited my old school, Rustenburg, and gazed at the oh so familiar buildings set against the backdrop of Devils Peak and the eastern ramparts of Table Mountain. At the University Ballet School I was welcomed by the new generation of dancers, who with their leotards and neat, scraped back ballet buns brought an acute pang of nostalgia to my heart.

I went further up Devils Peak to the main University, to the old ivy covered Psychology building which had been my father's second home. Down in Wynberg I tried in vain to find the old roller-skating rink. Later I gazed in tearful wonder at the long swathes of green turf at Kenilworth Race Course. I could almost hear the thunder of hooves, remembering the excitement of riding in amateur Ladies races. I drove to all my old haunts, gasping at the beauty of the Cape Peninsula which as a child I had taken for granted. And wherever I went, there was glorious Table Mountain, guiding me like a beacon and reminding me of my youth.

On my way back north to Zambia I stopped to see old friends in Johannesburg, and while we were sitting on their patio in the Frangipani fragrant cool of the evening, the phone rang.

It was Colin for me.

At first I didn't understand what he was saying. I had forgotten Andrew's check-up that morning. Julie was going with him and I hadn't been at all worried about the outcome. Then Colin's words began to percolate my brain.

"The lump is much bigger ... they're going to remove it ... to see whether it is malignant or not ..."

I froze.

Poor Andrew. Just when it had seemed his life was beginning again. And here was I, thousands of miles away ...

"I'll go as soon as I can," I told Colin.

- 0 -

Back in Lusaka I tipped the summer clothes from my suitcase and filled it with winter ones. Then I booked the first seat I could get to the UK. Dr Jelliffe had agreed the operation could be done at The Christie Hospital in Manchester, one of the major cancer hospitals in England, instead of at The Middlesex. At least I would not have the problem of London accommodation.

That night there was an excited call from Andrew.

"I didn't get the B Cal job but I've just had the interview with American Airlines. I'm sure I'll get it. Training in Dallas. All the airline perks. And a fantastic salary!" Not a word about the lump or the forthcoming operation at The Christie. He was focused on getting a job and that was all that seemed to matter.

We wished him luck and I said I'd see him in a couple of days.

It sounded too good to be true, but I was worried he might not get the job. And I was puzzled. Would he go on being rejected forever? I was certain he was being discriminated against. Was nobody prepared to take a chance on him? Were these people acting legitimately, or were they breaking the law? Was there a law?

I boarded the plane in Lusaka in a relatively relaxed state of mind. Everything is relative, I told myself, and he'd been through worse. But if the lump was malignant, what would happen next? Wasn't it a waste of time even thinking of looking for a job?

Only time would tell.

- 0 -

In the shuttle lounge at Heathrow I sit waiting for my connection to Manchester. It's too early for breakfast so I settle for a cup of hot tea in a plastic mug. How weird air transport is, the way it picks you up and dumps you down so quickly in another world.

It had been snowing, and through the big plate glass windows I gaze at the airfield stretching out in front of me like a giant skating rink. As it turns from dark grey to pinkish white, I am skating away on the icy expanse, skating towards the sun where a new day is dawning; and I know that I must keep skating, that I must never stop, and that at the end it will be a wonderful sight that I will see.

It will be Andrew. Completely well. I can see him there already.

Smiling.

Unblemished.

Perfect.

- 0 -

From the window of the Tri-Star the countryside was ninety percent white, the streets, rivers and houses like a grey tapestry woven into the blanket of snow. As we descended, Manchester shimmered in the first weak rays of sunshine.

I buttoned up my winter coat.

Peter was there to meet me. Good, reliable, dependable, lovable

236

Peter. He hoisted my suitcase into the boot of the car.

"Andrew is seeing the oncology specialist at The Christie on Wednesday," he told me as we drove off. "He's very apprehensive about the operation but he's being very sensible about it."

Sensible. I nodded, wondering what that meant, thinking to myself that sensible was hardly the word to use for the quality which had seen Andrew through this whole ghastly thing and which hopefully would see him through this next trauma too.

I think Andrew secretly enjoyed having me with him again. Fresh orange juice at his bedside in the morning, a sandwich for his lunch break, dinner hot and steaming on the table when he came home. Not to mention ironed shirts and underpants and matching pairs of socks.

The day after I arrived he asked me to type some job application letters. "Here's a draft letter, Mum, and a list of all the airlines in the country. I can't count on American Airlines," he added wistfully.

There were over twenty letters. Nothing was going to stop him now.

- 0 -

The Christie Hospital was a surprise. The décor was quietly elegant, the wall to wall carpet a soft shade of duck egg blue, the music suitable for a quickstep. Nobody looked miserable and there were no queues.

Bemused, we sat down in the soft comfortable chairs in the waiting area. Andrew leaned towards me and said in his best airport voice: "Pan-Am Airlines announces the arrival of their flight A1 from Honolulu," and we both laughed. It was so different from the big London teaching hospitals with their scrubbed floors and dingy dullness.

In a warm, pleasant consulting room Andrew undressed. A moment later a tall young doctor with bright red hair came in, smiling. Andrew was uneasy about seeing new doctors but this one made him feel very much at ease. After a thorough examination he said the lump had to be removed, but mainly because of Andrew's medical history. When the senior consultant arrived, he confirmed this.

He then saw the surgeon, whose quiet reserved manner also inspired him with confidence.

"Come in on Wednesday and we'll remove the lump on Thursday," he said. "It will then be examined under a microscope and we'll let you

237

know the results as soon as possible."

A week? Ten days? I wondered. Like last time ...

Andrew and I looked at each other. We had been there before. We'd bought the T-shirt.

Andrew then astounded me.

"I'd like it done under the NHS," he announced boldly.

"Why?" we all asked. He was covered by two private medical insurance companies, and at The Christie one had a choice.

Quick as a flash he answered. "Because if I have to have chemo again I want to be in a big ward where I can see other people with the same thing as me. And where I can see the nurses and they can see me."

I realised he'd been facing up to this all along. He was prepared for it. Prepared for the very worst, and I wanted to take him in my arms and hug him for his courage.

After that everything happened so quickly and efficiently and amiably that there was no time for Andrew to be apprehensive or frightened. Blood tests and chest X-rays were completed in minutes by this pleasant band of dedicated people who had made it their mission to treat cancer patients – or suspected cancer patients – in such a way that they did not feel as though they were entering the condemned cell.

We left the hospital and Andrew went straight back to work. I carried on typing the letters to the airlines. I was glad he had his travel agency job even though it gave him little satisfaction, for at least it got him out of bed in the morning and helped to keep his mind off the forthcoming operation.

- 0 -

On Thursday everything went smoothly. He was out of theatre in just over an hour and appeared to be in very little pain. He made none of the expected fuss and I thought how quickly he had grown up. The hospital was very close to our flat so I visited several times a day and so did Julie. Sometimes I picked her up and we had a chance to talk. I had the feeling that she loved him very much.

It would be a week before the pathology results were known.

Even though everyone from Philip down had told Andrew the lump was unlikely to be a malignant growth because that wasn't the usual pattern of osteosarcoma, none of us fully appreciated that this was because osteosarcoma cells are spread through the blood stream and not through the lymphatic system.

Yet, although we had all tried to feel optimistic about the result, there was still an agonising doubt. Why else would Mr Sweetnam and Dr Jelliffe and the doctors at The Christie have decided on an investigation?

On the morning after the operation the surgeon visited Andrew.

"The gland was very big," he reported solemnly.

Andrew didn't like the sound of that and neither did I. But he looks too well, I told myself; too positive, too full of life for anything sinister to be wrong.

He was discharged on Friday afternoon.

"Why are you limping," I asked as we walked to the car.

"If you had stitches where I've got stitches, Mum, you'd be limping too!"

Apart from that and a bit of drowsiness left over from the anaesthetic, he seemed fine.

Colin arrived from Zambia the following morning. Waiting for the results would be a time when we needed to be together. Wednesday was an eternity away.

Chapter Twenty-five

March – April 1986

Every day letters were arriving from the airlines to which Andrew had written. Not one offered him an interview. Some said they would put his application on their files but I did not believe them.

With no word yet from American Airlines he decided to phone them. "So sorry," they said. "You were unsuccessful." Perhaps Jo was right in wanting him to delay looking for a job, but he had the bit between his teeth and in spite of this new disappointment he carried on hoping.

- 0 -

When we got out of bed on Monday morning there was no way we could have guessed what a momentous week this would be for Andrew.

That evening on TV, Singapore Airlines with their swish new aircraft and exotic dark-eyed hostesses was splashed all over the screen, plugging their new flights direct from Manchester to Australia.

Andrew's alert blue eyes drew together in a puzzled frown. "I didn't get a reply from Singapore Airlines, did I, Mum?"

Mentally I skimmed through the rejections. "No. I wonder why."

"Right. I'll ring them tomorrow."

"I'm sorry," the manager said. "We've completed our recruitment programme."

"Thank you," Andrew replied, and slammed down the phone.

The disappointment and frustration boiled up inside him. Then he breathed in deeply and let the air out slowly, tipping his head back until he was looking at the ceiling.

"Am I ever going to get a job?"

That afternoon I escaped to the city centre, leaving Andrew and his Dad watching television. I had to stop thinking about tomorrow's pathology result and shopping was as good a way to blank my mind as any.

I stayed out as long as I could, knowing how waiting for news could stretch time beyond its limits. When I finally returned I popped my head into the lounge to say hello. The two of them looked at me in a peculiar way.

"We've got some bad news," Andrew said.

I dropped my parcels. The blood drained from my head. We were only supposed to get news about the lump tomorrow, so what on earth was all this about?

Andrew got up quickly and put his arms around me. "It's okay, Mum. Only pulling your leg. The hospital phoned. There's nothing wrong with me. Really!"

"Oh you ... you rotten –"

They were both grinning from ear to ear and I didn't know whether to laugh or cry.

Straight away we phoned Philip and Jo and all the family and close friends to tell them the wonderful news, and I kept pinching myself to make sure it hadn't all been a dream.

- 0 -

I was learning that tragedy and suffering somehow seem to put things into perspective. Without them the good things would seem ordinary, routine, dull. Next morning I danced into the kitchen to squeeze the orange juice, thinking how privileged I was to know how extraordinarily wonderful the good things could be.

Just before breakfast there was a call for Andrew.

I heard him say "Hello".

A couple of minutes later he rushed into the kitchen. "He wants me to come for an interview! Tomorrow! At two o'clock!"

"Who?"

"The manager of Singapore Airlines!"

Breathless with excitement he searched for an atlas and anything else that would tell him about Singapore and Australia. I dashed into town, to the airline's Manchester office and grabbed every leaflet I could lay my hands on so that he could learn as much as possible before his interview.

He didn't sleep a wink that night. I heard him walking around, saw

241

his light go on and off. I lay staring at the ceiling, haunted by visions of yet another rejection. I wanted to take him away from it all. Now. To Menorca or Zambia or anywhere far enough away from people who could be so cruel to him.

Next day, still grey with lack of sleep, Andrew got dressed in the pale grey suit.

"Do I look the part, Dad?"

Together they decided it wasn't quite right and he changed into grey trousers and his smart new navy blue blazer.

I smiled at him. "The perfect airline man," I said, though I knew that appearances alone never got anyone a job. He would also have to be good.

"I've got to get this job, Mum. I've just got to get it."

I rushed around the flat doing my chores, pleading silently: *Please give him this chance. Please. Please. Please.*

- 0 -

It was a freezing cold day. We parked in the Arndale Centre, then hovered in and out of Marks and Spencer to keep warm, not taking our eyes off the doors of the glass fronted building in Shambles Square through which Andrew, still with the stitches in his groin, had limped; not wanting to miss the moment when he walked out.

Two-thirty. Two forty-five. Three. Still no sign of Andrew.

"A long interview is a good sign," Colin said, squeezing my arm.

At five past three he appeared.

We ran towards him. I linked my arm in his and Colin moved in on his other side.

His face was heavy with dejection. "I'll never get that job," he said.

I felt a surge of anger. "Why the hell not?"

"Not enough experience."

We went home, silent and despondent. I cooked supper. We tried to watch television. Nothing cheered him up. Colin made some cocoa and handed him a cup.

"Remember what Uncle Stan always says, son, that it's all right to smile and be cheerful?"

"Yes, but tell me again." Uncle Stan was his idol.

Colin repeated his brother's favourite rhyme and as usual Andrew burst out laughing. I laughed too because Andrew's laugh is so infectious.

"Yes. You're right, Dad. I suppose there is still a faint chance."

Maybe, but I had my doubts. Singapore Airlines would be just like all the others. They would reject him and already I hated them.

- 0 -

I flicked open a corner of the curtain; it was dark and grey and wet and freezing cold, a good morning for a lie-in with the papers. I snuggled back into bed and just then the phone rang. Through our open door we heard Andrew answer it from the extension next to his bed.

"Hello," he said. "Yes. Speaking. What? *Fantastic!* Yes! When do you want me to start? Thank you. Thank you very very much!"

As we leapt out of bed Andrew flew into our room.

"I've got the job! I've got the job! I can't believe it. I've got a proper job!"

Everyone was happy for Andrew. Especially Julie, who was always around these days. "I'm proud of him," she said that evening in her sweet, quiet voice, her blue eyes shining with love.

A letter arrived on Monday from the Singapore Airlines head office in London confirming their offer. Andrew handed it to me to read.

"What's wrong, Mum?"

A sentence had jumped out from the page. I read it to him.

"... subject to a medical examination by an independent authority ..."

What cruel twist was this?

Would his medical history prevent him from getting this job too? Would they give it to him with one hand and take it away with the other? Would they be as heartless as the banks had been?

Would it all happen again?

"Not a problem, Mum. It's only routine. Anyway, I'm perfectly fit. There's not a thing wrong with me."

The medical examination was due to take place in London during Andrew's probationary training period at the airline's London headquarters – on the very day we were flying back to Lusaka.

We always seemed to be flying somewhere and sometimes I longed to stay in one place.

- 0 -

We flew to Heathrow, collected our luggage and wheeled it through the maze of passages and walk-ways to Terminal Three. We sat in the departure lounge feeling pretty glum. How utterly excruciating to have to leave without knowing the result of the medical.

Please let him get through it, I pleaded silently. *Maybe they won't notice he has a leg full of metal, and will ignore his history of cancer. Surely they wouldn't let him get this far and then turn him down?*

I looked at my watch. We'd be boarding any minute but just then we heard a voice booming over the loudspeakers.

"That was for us!" I said to Colin, whose nose was buried in a flying magazine. "Asking us to report to Information!"

We hurried to the desk. The BA girl gave the phone to Colin. It was Andrew, phoning from the Singapore Airlines office upstairs in this same enormous building.

"No problems, Dad. I'm through the medical. But I'm afraid I have no airport authority yet to enter the departure lounge, so I can't see you."

We told him we loved him, and still walking on air, we boarded our plane.

Just before taking off the hostess filled our glasses with Champagne. We clinked them together. "To Andrew," Colin said.

I smiled. Too choked up to speak.

- O -

Every night for weeks I lay outside on our dew-covered lawn and watched Halley's Comet. Clearly visible in Zambia's dry-season cloudless skies, its tail was a furry blob of mist traversing the vast Milky Way.

Soon it would be gone, not to appear again for another seventy years. I wouldn't be around, but was fascinated by the thought that Andrew might just make it.

It seemed his ordeal was over. He had struggled to overcome his illness, fought back to make a new and different life. He had never given up, and as one door closed he made another one open.

He had become a different person, with new values and ideals; he had become more thoughtful and considerate, and more aware of other people's problems. On the way he had sacrificed the things he

244

had most loved to do, the things he had considered important. But what, I wondered sadly, had happened to his dreams?

Chapter Twenty-six

1986 – 1989

While our two other sons, Colin and Peter, were forging ahead with their careers, Andrew was now on the first rung of his career as an airline man. Peter was making a name for himself as a criminal defence lawyer, and Colin, having left Zambia in March 1985 when his first wife was tragically diagnosed with MS and needed treatment in the UK, was now at the South Crofty tin mine in Cornwall, working his way up the promotional ladder and appointed Mine Superintendent in 1989.

For Andrew, a decade younger than his brothers, it would be a slower progress. At first it was exciting working for Singapore Airlines. The training in Singapore for his job as a reservation and ticketing agent was an adventure in itself and there were holidays with Julie in exotic places like Penang, Tenerife, Florida and the Maldives – that cluster of tropical coral atolls in the Indian Ocean where the transparent turquoise waters first lured him to scuba-diving.

Further trips to Singapore followed for more advanced training. Singapore Airlines was voted Best Airline of the Year in 1987 and it seemed there could never be a dull moment.

But soon the routine job, well mastered after a couple of years, with certificates of competence and letters of appreciation from satisfied customers, was not enough to satisfy Andrew's thirst for challenge.

Even the rifle shooting, at which he now excelled, seemed slightly jaded, especially without the inspiration of Uncle Stan who sadly died suddenly in late 1986. It was as though Andrew had to prove to himself not only that he was no different from anyone else, nor in any way a misfit, but that he was capable of doing anything he set his mind to. Because his life was threatened he had an even bigger hunger for life than before.

To satisfy this growing appetite he took up Scuba Diving. He was already swimming regularly as a means of keeping fit, but swimming was tame and boring compared to diving for sunken treasure. A year later he passed the British Sub Aqua examinations, but good dives were few and far between in Britain's coastal waters: a far cry from the sparkling seas of the Maldives and the Canaries.

Then in 1988 something happened to change his life.

- 0 -

It is Sunday morning and we are wading through *The Times* and *The Telegraph* and *The Sunday Mail*. I am in the kitchen making coffee when I hear Andrew shout.

"Dad. Look at this! British Airways. They're going to train pilots!"

At first it's just the BA advert itself that is a challenge, taunting him. It's their first pilot training scheme for over a decade and in the end he can't possibly ignore it when it's splashed across every national newspaper for weeks on end.

He applies.

Not a surprise, really, for though we never speak about the lost flying career, nobody can forget that Andrew had first decided to be a pilot at the age of eight, and that at seventeen the RAF had offered him that prestigious Flying Scholarship.

Peter tries to dissuade him.

"Okay, Peter," Andrew says impatiently. "I know my leg will stop me getting in but if I don't try I'll never know for sure, will I? And I'd hate to spend the rest of my life kicking myself because I didn't give it a go."

What I like is his amazing capacity for taking risks. Cast in the same mould as his father he is not prepared to remain cocooned in the confines of a safe, easy life. He knows that if he doesn't attempt to stretch himself beyond that ease, he will never know what he is really capable of.

In his carefully worded letter of application he explains his medical history, along with his life-long passion to fly.

They send him an application form. A pilot friend tells us they only send forms to a fraction of the thousands of applicants. He knows, because his son has not received one back.

Andrew's hopes double. He sends off the form. Secretly I think outright rejection at this stage wouldn't be a bad thing.

Seven days pass.

On the eighth day a letter plops through the slot in the door. Feverishly Andrew opens it. "Come for an interview," they say, and inwardly I groan.

The interview goes well; and miracle of miracles, he is selected for flying aptitude tests.

His anticipation soars, for already he has passed with distinction similar tests at Biggin Hill, his success proven by the RAF's doomed offer of the scholarship.

We phone Peter to tell him the news. "He'll never get in," he says. "Why don't you stop him now, before it's too late?"

I laugh. "Stop him? Impossible! Besides, it would be cruel to dampen his enthusiasm now, when he's got so far."

"Well," Peter says, "I just hope his growing ability to take knocks and disappointments will cushion him against the final blow."

Peter has taken the words out of my mouth. The five year period is not up yet. There's still one year to go before he can be deemed a survivor from cancer, and I still worry about the effects of stress.

He gets through the aptitude tests.

He is jubilant. Colin and I are very proud, though we know the final step is crucial – the medical examination.

His amazing success so far in the selection process has refuelled the fires of his burning desire to fly, and with his hopes literally sky-high he goes for the examination. In the excruciatingly slow days that follow, no one dares speculate on the result.

At last comes the day of reckoning.

It is a Monday. The postman is late and the letter arrives after Andrew has left for work. I phone Peter and Andrea, and catch Julie at the office and ask them all to gather at the house this evening to help soften the blow when Andrew comes home.

There is dead silence. No-one breathes. He opens the letter. We hear the exaggerated crackle of paper as he reads it through.

I bite my bottom lip to keep it from trembling, but Andrew puts us all at ease with a little half smile that turns up the corners of his mouth.

He reads it once more. Silently.

Then slowly he looks up.

"Well, you lot. At least I know for certain now. I'll never fly."

He folds up the letter and places it in the envelope.

He smiles again.

248

"I'm glad I gave it a go."

- 0 -

But the seeds of change had been sewn. Though for a while he settled down, he constantly complained that working on the third floor of a city centre office block was not his idea of a career in the airline industry, and whenever he had the chance to work overtime at the airport, he did so.

We had by this time left Zambia for good, Colin having retired early from the Zambian mining industry in order to be nearer Andrew. We had moved to our house in Menorca and had sold the flat in Manchester and bought a house in Cheshire, where Andrew now lived. We both felt happier being closer to England. We could fly there in just over two hours if we were suddenly needed. Not that we thought this would ever be necessary: the longed for figure of five years was fast approaching, when Andrew would be considered cured.

Besides he never mentioned his leg these days.

Never mentioned pain.

Never even hinted that it had begun to swell up.

- 0 -

Soon after his holiday with Julie in Florida at the beginning of 1989, he phoned us in Menorca.

"What do you think about air-traffic control, Dad?"

"It's a stressful job. Why?"

"I want to be at the sharp end, Dad. If I can't fly, why can't I be an air traffic control officer in the RAF? What do you think? Shall I go for it?"

What could Colin say?

"Of course, son, if that's what you want. But what makes you think you'll get through the medical?"

"My leg won't be a problem, Dad. Air traffic control is a sedentary job."

"But Andrew, all officers in the RAF have to be A1 fit, no matter what they do."

We flew to England to plan our long awaited holiday to New Zealand and Australia, and just before we left, Andrew got a reply from

249

the RAF. They sent him an application form and he returned it, full of hope and confidence.

"I'm sure I'll get this, Dad," he said as we were packing for our twelve thousand mile trip to Christchurch. "They're short of controllers and I have all the pre-qualifications they need."

He still didn't mention the painful, swollen leg.

"But if you got in, Andrew, you'd be an officer, and RAF officers have to do routine marching and go on manoeuvres and all that stuff."

"Yes, Dad. I know. But I'm sure they'll make an exception."

He got an interview. Then a letter inviting him for a further interview. Meanwhile they had read his medical history on the form and were requesting a detailed report from Mr Sweetnam.

- 0 -

When we got back from our grand trip to New Zealand and Oz there was a large discoloured lump on Andrew's leg which he could no longer hide. He'd been to The Christie Hospital for X-rays but had not yet received a report as this would be sent directly to The Middlesex.

Two days later I went with him up to London. Mr Sweetnam was surprised to see him so soon. Only at the beginning of January he had told him not to come back for one whole year.

I was glad I decided to go with him. He had said, "No, Mum. Don't worry. I'll be fine on my own." But thank goodness I insisted.

It was just short of the magical five years.

- 0 -

The doors slide open at Goodge Street Underground station. Memories of five years ago flood back. I recall the horror as I re-trace my steps into the hospital forecourt, through the swing doors, past the rows of chairs and down the passage to Mr Sweetnam's domain.

Nothing seems to have changed.

"Now, what's the problem, Andrew?" Mr Sweetnam asks in his usual lively manner.

Andrew hesitates a moment. "Well, sir, I've got this swelling on my leg."

He does not mention the pain.

Mr Sweetnam frowns. "Where?"

250

Andrew lifts his trouser leg. The swelling is monstrous.

"Hmm. Well, let's have a look at you. Bend your knee, Andrew. That's very good," he says. "Now lift the leg up straight."

Andrew lifts it. He turns his head away to hide the pain. But not so that I don't see it.

"Excellent. Now let's see you walk."

Andrew walks across the room and back again.

"He walks very well, doesn't he?" Mr Sweetnam says, pleased with his creation.

"Yes," I answer, equally pleased and remembering the day long ago when he'd said Andrew would always limp.

Mr Sweetnam rubs his chin as he leafs through the report from The Christie Hospital about the X-rays.

"Now, I'd really like to X-ray this leg again, Andrew, to see what's causing the swelling, but you had X-rays three weeks ago at The Christie, didn't you. We can't do it again so soon."

"No, sir."

"So I'll ask The Christie to lend me the X-rays."

Suddenly Andrew leans forward.

"Mr Sweetnam —" His voice is charged with urgency.

Mr Sweetnam raises his eyebrows, his dictaphone still at his mouth.

"Could you please write to the RAF. They want a report on my leg."

Mr Sweetnam's eyes open wide as Andrew explains about his application to become an RAF air traffic control officer.

He puts down his dictaphone.

"The less I write to them, you know, Andrew, the better." He pauses. "I wouldn't suggest it for a minute."

Andrew's mouth slowly drops open.

Mr Sweetnam glances down at Andrew's leg. He takes a deep breath. "I could give them a straight description of the operation we did in 1984," he goes on, "but right now ..." He shakes his head. "Right now the less we say about it, the better."

He looks directly at Andrew. In his eyes a rare betrayal of tenderness is fleetingly unmasked, before the skin stretches taut again over the long fine bones of his expressive face.

"They won't take you, you know, Andrew. It would be impossible to get in."

I watch closely for Andrew's reaction and my chest tightens as I see yet another dream shatter into tiny pieces.

251

Then suddenly I realise what this visit is all about.

He isn't really bothered about his painful leg and the enormous swelling. This is only about persuading Mr Sweetnam to write a favourable letter to the RAF in reply to their request!

Mr Sweetnam carries on talking into his dictaphone. Suddenly Andrew puts his head in his hands as though he feels unwell, and in the jumble of the words which follow we hear the word *amputation*.

Mr Sweetnam does a double take. His lean face creases with surprise. The pretty blonde Sister in attendance stands rock still.

"Good heavens!" Mr Sweetnam says. "Who said anything about amputation? There are a thousand things I'd do before that."

Andrew stares at Mr Sweetnam.

"Andrew ... don't worry," he says firmly. "You've survived cancer. Just remember that. First and foremost you've survived cancer and that outweighs everything else. You're alive! Just think about it, and tell yourself you're alive. And because you're alive you're able to worry."

He pauses for a moment. "And then tell yourself you've got your leg." His voice softens. "If you hadn't come to us when you did, you wouldn't have it. They would have cut it off and that would have been that. And you'd have gone on with your life without a leg."

Yes, I think to myself, *if it hadn't been for Philip ...*

This is the most impassioned speech we've ever heard from Mr Sweetnam. I was wrong five years ago to assume that Dr Jelliffe was the only one concerned about Andrew's quality of life. It seems Mr Sweetnam has always been just as concerned.

"No! The last thing I'd do is amputate your leg," he says, becoming quite emotional for Mr Sweetnam, who is usually so totally down-to-earth.

But something he said must have triggered off the thought of amputation in Andrew's head. I know he'll bounce back by the end of the day, the way he always does, but right now he looks extremely upset.

"Come and see me in a month, Andrew, and we'll do a CT scan on the same day. By then we'll have the X-rays from The Christie. At the same time I'll take some of that fluid off." He points to the swollen leg.

Andrew looks alarmed at the mention of taking fluid off.

It means a needle.

Mr Sweetnam goes on talking into his dictaphone. Suddenly he looks up again. "On second thoughts, we'll ask The Christie to do the CT scan." He runs back the tape and rephrases his letter to The Christie.

I watch with awe this dynamic man as his course of action evolves. You can almost see his mind flashing, both through the changes of expression in his dark brown eyes and the way the planes of his face flex and mould around his thoughts. For a moment he is still, then he erupts into action again.

"No." He shakes his head. "We can't wait to take off that fluid. We'd better do it right now."

Andrew cringes. His face drains to an opaline whiteness. His head sinks onto his chest. A moment later he lifts it again as he resolves to accept Mr Sweetnam's new plan but I can see that he is still badly shaken by the threat of amputation.

I remember how it was five years ago when he was afraid it would rob him of his masculinity. But now there is a new dimension to his fear.

The RAF would never take a man with only one leg.

Not even to be an air traffic controller.

He looks searchingly at Mr Sweetnam.

"But everything has been so good," he says, trying to regain his composure. "And now ... *this!*" There is despair in his voice.

"It still *is* good, Andrew," Mr Sweetnam says firmly. "But until I see the X-rays I can't do any more. I can't X-ray you today so we won't make any firm appointment to see you again until I've heard from The Christie."

The pretty blonde Sister leads us out and asks us to wait in the corridor outside the treatment rooms. The last forty minutes have been emotionally draining for me, but for Andrew it has been hell. He turns to me as we sit down.

"I'm glad you came with me, Mum."

I nod, my lips pressed into a tight smile as I try to keep my face from breaking into a contortion of emotion. "Yes." I squeeze his hand, wishing I could do something to reassure him. "But I don't know what Mr Sweetnam said that made you think he would amputate your leg. You over-reacted, Andrew. You can't expect him to write a letter saying your leg is okay when it obviously isn't."

Mr Sweetnam's words echo in my ears. *They won't take you, you know, Andrew. It would be impossible to get in.*

Andrew buries his face in his hands. "I know him well, Mum. He didn't look happy."

"You misunderstood him. Of course he's concerned but I'm sure it's something he'll be able to fix." I slide my arm around his shoulder, and just then the Sister asks him to go into the treatment room.

Curtains are drawn around the cubicle and he gets undressed again. I hear him exclaim softly as the needle is inserted. Mr Sweetnam fills a container with the fluid so that it can be analysed and five minutes later Andrew appears ashen-faced at the door.

In a delayed reaction to the needle he sways, his eyes roll back and he almost faints. I hold him up, steer him to a chair. The receptionist calls the pretty blonde Sister, and like the little green-eyed Sister from Greenhow Ward, she kneels in front of him. "Keep your head down between your legs, Andrew. You're in the best possible hands, you know."

"Yes," Andrew says, his voice barely audible. "I know I am. He's brilliant. I know that." He puts his head down again. "But I'm *not* going to let him take my leg. I won't let him!"

"He won't do that," Sister says softly. "You heard him, Andrew."

"I won't let him," he insists, like someone demented.

A little colour returns to his cheeks. Everything she says is so logical that he is finally persuaded he'd been wrong. I see the exact moment when he is truly convinced; there is a kind of relaxation in the muscles of his face, though the shock of his misapprehension takes longer to dissipate.

Finally it's time for him to go for the blood test. He shows no sign of the old fear, though he still looks as though he can't believe he is back at The Middlesex, under threat of yet another operation.

As we go out into the sunshine I tell him how impressed I am that he withstood the needle without flinching.

"Oh, I'm not worried any more about them sticking needles into me for blood tests, Mum. It's only having a needle in my leg and maybe infecting it that worries me. It's okay as it is. Nothing must contaminate it."

We'd both been told long ago how vital it was that no infection should ever invade the hallowed inner areas of the prosthesis; and that such a contamination might prove impossible to eradicate because of the difficulty of antibiotics finding their way to the hidden recesses where the bone merges with the alien metal of the prosthesis, where

254

few or no blood vessels exist for their passage; and that such an infection might prove fatal to the continued existence of the prosthesis.

"There's no chance of that," I assure him, knowing how precious his leg is to him but realising that his somewhat paranoiac reaction this afternoon has left him with an unrealistic fear and suspicion.

"Mr Sweetnam will have taken every precaution possible."

"Yes, of course he will. I know that, Mum."

Mr Sweetnam wasn't the Queen's Surgeon for nothing.

Chapter Twenty-seven

1989 – 1991

Andrew dragged the long, tight elastic stocking over his leg.

"I am not going to let this swelling get any worse," he said, going to the corner of the lounge where he kept his cello. "And I'm not going to let the pain take over my life."

He took the cover off the cello and the sunlight shafting through the window caught the rich russet glow of the wood. "I wish I knew what was wrong," he said angrily. "The result of the tests showed no infection. The X-rays showed nothing either. So what the hell is going on?"

"I wish I knew, Andrew. But just keep on thinking positively."

I listened to the discordant notes as he tuned the instrument and a moment later a flood of bitter-sweet anguish flowed from his bow. The rich resonance rustled through my body, touching every nerve end as the plaintive melody rose to a crescendo of passion that gushed from his inner soul.

We were all baffled, including Mr Sweetnam, and it was a stressful time for Andrew. Next to his bed was a copy of the Simonton's book about learning to relax and visualise recovery, much of which was similar to the methods I had learnt from the foot reflexology lady. He was often able to control the pain this way, but the cello seemed to do it more effectively.

Control the pain, yes; but not the swelling. The swelling got worse. So at the end of May he was admitted to The Middlesex for a biopsy in order to determine what was going on.

The surgeons opened up the leg. They had a good look around. They removed all the fluid and the inflamed tissue and found that the bone surrounding the spike of the titanium prosthesis had begun to erode away.

There was a small cavity where before there had been bone. Unbelievably, it looked as though it was only a residue of cement that

256

was holding everything precariously together.

This sounded serious, and once again we were living on the edge of an abyss while we waited for laboratory results.

The results were negative. No infection. Nothing. At least that was one hurdle cleared.

Yet clearly *something* was happening. Precisely what, nobody knew. Except that for some reason the bone wasn't happy with the presence of the metal.

Was it being rejected, I wondered.

A week later Andrew was discharged, with yet another stern warning from Mr Sweetnam to take it easy.

"No long walks, Andrew. And no carrying heavy weights."

He recovered quickly and was soon back at work. Colin and I flew back to Menorca where we played golf and swam in the sea and soaked up the sun. We phoned Andrew every Sunday and for a while everything was fine.

Then at the beginning of November there was a change.

- 0 -

Three things happened.

The leg began to swell again. It looked angry and red, and two little black spots appeared near the site of the recent biopsy. I said I would fly over but he wouldn't hear of it.

The following week he and Julie decided to call off their five-year long relationship. They were still fond of each other, Andrew said, but it wasn't working out. I think the problem was that she wanted to get married and start a family, whereas Andrew was nowhere near ready for this. I was sad that it had ended. She'd been so good for him. I could tell that he was upset and now I wanted even more to fly over, but still he would not hear of it.

Each Sunday when we phoned we could only take his word that the leg was no worse.

Agonising over his aloneness I wondered whether the umbilical cord is ever really cut. Whether one can ever totally sever the seemingly infrangible bond that exists between mother and child. When do children cease to need their parents' help? When are they no longer children? Andrew was twenty-four now, but I still felt responsible for his well-being.

257

The third thing that happened was that Andrew decided he was going to fly an aeroplane.

Everything else receded into the background. We stopped hearing about his leg and heard instead about his adventurous plans.

He knew that nobody would ever sponsor him to fly, and to obtain a British Private Pilot Licence was completely beyond his financial means. He had been saving up ever since joining Singapore Airlines but this money wouldn't even cover half the fees.

But in South Africa he could get his training for half the cost.

He had four weeks leave due and booked this for January, when the weather in the Cape would be perfect. As one of his airline perks he bought a return air ticket to Johannesburg for ten percent of the normal fare.

"What about his leg?" I asked Colin one Sunday afternoon after the latest phone update on Andrew's plans. "How will he manage?"

Colin looked at me wryly. The leg hadn't been mentioned for weeks. "Don't worry. I'm sure Mr Sweetnam won't let him go before he gets rid of the swelling and those ominous black spots. Besides, this is all just part of his old dream to fly, which he can't let go of. It'll all fizzle out ..."

Andrew only seemed worried about two things.

First, his check-up on the twenty-second of December when it was highly likely Mr Sweetnam would admit him straight away because his leg had deteriorated so much.

And second, the South Africans were insisting the flying medical examination be done in South Africa. They would not accept a British medical certificate.

Ignoring this Andrew had a test done by Dr Ian Donnan at Manchester Airport. He passed. It was only a Class 3 medical, the minimum required by the CAA for a UK Private Pilot Licence, but he was jubilant.

"The South Africans can't possibly fail me now, can they Dad?"

Colin and I returned to England for Christmas. Andrew could talk of nothing else but the forthcoming flying course. I still believed that something would stop him going but I also prayed that he would go, because he wanted this more than anything he had ever wanted in his life.

He insisted on gong alone for his check-up just before Christmas. He said he would go by air rather than by train or car. He was probably afraid I would make too much fuss and influence Mr Sweetnam's decision. When I looked at the leg that morning I couldn't see how Mr Sweetnam would allow him to go. The swelling was enormous. It was red and blue and purple. The black dots had grown to saucer size, so big that they'd almost joined together. I wanted him to go to South Africa, yet I feared that something might happen to the leg while he was there. So much so that I took out extra BUPA insurance in case he needed to be flown back to England in an emergency.

That night we went to meet him at Manchester Airport on his return from London. People were streaming through the barrier. At last we saw him with his stick, hurrying towards us as fast as he could, without actually running.

We took one look at the broad grin and knew the news was good.

"Mr Sweetnam said I could go!"

How I loved that man for saying yes.

The car was just outside the terminal building. "Did you have to do a lot of persuading to make him let you go?" I asked as we drove off into the cold wet night. I knew how persuasive Andrew could be.

"No, I didn't," he said with an innocent smile. "He was very encouraging. But he said, *Be very careful.*"

His life-long dream was within his grasp.

Julie had left a big gap in his life and I knew he still missed her, but right now nothing could have filled that gap better than this.

In the few days left before his departure for South Africa he rested the leg whenever he could, strapped it up tightly and used a walking stick wherever he went.

He was taking no chances.

All arrangements were made. The finances were taken care of with every penny of his savings. He had an appointment for his flying medical test in Pretoria two days after his arrival. He would then fly down to Port Alfred. To his El Dorado. His *raison d'être.*

To 43 Air School.

- O -

He boarded the plane to Johannesburg on New Year's Eve – a good time to fly he told me, as most people were already at their holiday destinations. Another good time was Christmas Eve, and of course, Friday the thirteenth. With the predictable three seats to himself he

259

kept the leg up all night during the twelve hour flight.

So far so good; but in Pretoria the doctor giving him the flying medical test had just had a heart attack. No other doctor could fit him in at short notice.

Andrew was frantic. With no medical he could not embark on the course.

Finally, on the day before the start of his three week course, he managed to see an alternate doctor. He had waited almost a week.

"That wasn't all, Dad. When I arrived at 43 Air School they said I couldn't start flying until the actual medical certificate arrived from Pretoria. Then the next day the head of the school heard from Pretoria that there was a problem because of my leg and the history of cancer."

Andrew could see his dream evaporating in the thin cloudless air of Port Alfred.

"It's unbelievable!" he said. "They're insisting on a full medical report. And a scan!"

I wanted to scream. We were six thousand miles away with only a phone between us. There was nothing we could do. The thought of the months of preparation, the excitement, the anticipation, the expense, the long journey ...

In the end they reached a compromise: they gave him a temporary medical certificate to fly in South Africa for thirty days only.

"Thank goodness," Colin said. "That's just long enough for him to get his PPL."

Two days later he phoned again.

"I don't think I'm going to manage it, Mum."

"What do you mean?"

This was all he'd ever wanted to do and now he was telling me he didn't think he could do it! I went hot and cold as I waited for his answer.

"It's my leg."

I feared the worst.

"It just won't work. It's got no power. I can't work the plane's rudder pedals."

"Just keep trying, darling ..."

I thrust the phone into Colin's hand and went to make a pot of strong hot Rooibos tea.

Just keep trying ... I'm sure you can do it ... you must do it ...

Words, words, words ...

260

What bloody good were they when the bottom of Andrew's world was falling out?

A few minutes later Colin followed me into the kitchen. He shook his head and took me into his arms. I could feel his cheek wet on mine.

"A normal person doesn't even think about using his legs when flying an aeroplane," he said, still holding me tight. "I'd completely forgotten about the heavy rudder pedal pressures when taxiing a small aircraft, especially if it's windy."

I looked at him and sighed. "I think that's the most cruel blow of all."

"It will be a miracle if he makes it now."

Two days later, another phone call.

"Dad, the winds are blowing a gale."

The traditional South-Easters on that exposed southern coast were blowing with a vengeance. This made the rudder control even more difficult. To me, six thousand miles away and helpless, it seemed that everything was against him.

But he persevered.

As I suppose we knew he would.

With superhuman determination he devised a unique means of directing power from his hip and stomach muscles to his powerless knee.

It seemed slightly more hopeful now, but not much, since so much time had already been lost out of the scant three weeks.

"Well, at least he's giving it a go," Colin said resignedly.

"If he hadn't tried now, he'd always have wanted to, wouldn't he."

Colin's face twisted into a sad smile. "Yes. At least he's getting it out of his system. Even if he doesn't manage to go solo."

I looked at the wistful expression on my husband's face and smiled back. Finally, at the age of thirty-six, he'd had the opportunity to learn to fly and realise his own burning ambition, so he knew what he was talking about.

We were both living on a knife edge, willing Andrew to succeed.

I bit my lip until it hurt. "Wouldn't it be awful if he didn't get his PPL."

"It would be far worse if he didn't even succeed in going solo." Colin had a far-away look in his eyes. "Nothing can supplant the ecstasy of that first solo flight."

A few days later the phone rang again.

261

He had notched up ten hours of dual instruction flying.

"It's magic, Dad. Absolute magic. It's all I ever dreamed it would be. And much, much more."

Then there was a sadder note in his voice. "Two of the guys have already gone solo."

I couldn't imagine the instructors ever letting Andrew go solo if his leg wasn't strong enough to manage the rudder pedals easily. As much as I yearned for him to get his PPL, I had to be realistic.

Whatever will be, will be. Or, as we say in Menorca: *"Lo que serà, serà."*

On the twelfth day of the course, the phone rang.

The operator asked if I would pay the charges for a collect call from South Africa.

"Colin! Come quickly!" I yelled.

"What?"

"Someone calling from Port Alfred. I think something dreadful must have happened."

The line crackled. I heard a voice.

It was Andrew. He had run out of money!

"I've done it, Mum! I've gone solo!"

I could hardly speak. One moment it was as if I was standing in an ice cold shower. The next I was in a furnace. And then again in the cold shower.

In my bones I had known he would do it but there had been so many obstacles in his way.

"Fantastic, darling! So now you'll be able to get your PPL."

"Of course I will," he said, and my heart brimmed over with joy.

"Incredible," Colin whispered, wiping away a tear when he thought I wasn't looking.

Apart from the high cost of learning to fly in England, one other factor had led Andrew to do it in South Africa.

The weather.

January in the Cape Province is mid-summer, renowned for its cloudless blue skies.

But not so in January 1990. Oh no. Not only did the wind choose to blow harder than usual, but in the final week of the course the cloud came down over Port Alfred to a height of about one hundred feet.

Visibility was less than a mile. All flying was cancelled for two days – the two crucial days that were needed for Andrew to clock up the final two and a half hours he needed to get his licence.

You need forty hours and he had thirty-seven and a half.

"Sod's Law," Colin said, shaking his head with bitter disappointment.

This weather restriction affected nearly all the pupil pilots, but they were in a position to stay the extra day or two to complete the necessary hours. They wanted Andrew to do the same, but he was adamant.

"I have to get back to England. I must be at work on Wednesday. I've been away a month and they'll be short-handed if I don't get back on time. I can't let them down. Singapore Airlines have been so good to me."

"Phone them up and tell them you'll be late, Andy. Come on!" the other student pilots urged.

- 0 -

The long flight home from Port Alfred began on Sunday. He had done what he'd always wanted to do: he had learned to fly. He had gone solo. He didn't have the coveted Private Pilot's Licence, but he had something far more valuable. Something he was waiting to show us.

Something which had made it all worth while ...

- 0 -

We wait anxiously at the arrivals point at Manchester Airport.

"I'm so proud of him," Colin says, keeping his eye on the doors through which passengers are pouring. "It just doesn't matter that he hasn't got the licence. He can surely do the last few hours here in England anyway."

"Yes," I say dreamily. "The main thing is that he's done it. He has flown an aeroplane."

"And fantastic that his leg was okay in the end," Colin says, his eyes still glued to the doors where the stream of people is thinning out.

"He's taking a long time," I say impatiently.

Suddenly a BA official comes up to us.

"Are you Mr and Mrs Belshaw?"

My heart stands still.

Colin nods.

263

"Your son asked me to call you in. I'm afraid he's had a bit of an accident. It's his leg ..."

The guard on duty lets us through to the luggage collection area. Andrew's suitcase with its unmistakable red strap is going round and round the carousel, all on its own.

Then we see him.

He is lying on the floor, bent double. There is blood everywhere.

Frantically he holds up his leg, trying to stop the blood squirting from the huge swelling. He has already applied the sterile dressing Colin had insisted he take with him in case of just such an emergency. The twenty-three hour journey has taken its toll.

He says little and it's impossible to tell from his Spartan expression what is going on in his head.

Firemen appear with a wheel-chair. First Aid men apply another sterile dressing.

"I've been waiting for this to happen," he says as they wheel him to the airport doctor. "I've been expecting it."

The doctor takes one look. He telephones Withington Hospital to say he's sending Andrew straight to them and only then does Andrew realise the seriousness of what has happened.

At Withington Hospital the emergency doctor's face is grave. He orders X-rays and calls the orthopaedic consultant.

The consultant shakes his head. "The urgency lies in the danger which now exists for germs to enter through the punctured swollen area," he says. "With direct access to the bone."

An infection there, as we well know, might be catastrophic for Andrew's leg.

Three hours later we thank the caring doctor who admits frankly he has no idea how to proceed any further. He gives Andrew a powerful antibiotic and advises him to go at once to Mr Sweetnam.

As soon as we arrive home Andrew phones The Middlesex.

"Keep going with the antibiotics," the senior registrar tells him. "Keep the leg supported. Don't do any weight-bearing whatsoever on that leg. Come and see Mr Sweetnam on Friday and be prepared to be admitted immediately."

The next call is to Singapore Airlines to apologise for not being able to come back to work tomorrow. Ironic, when he'd sacrificed getting his PPL in order to be back on time.

The third thing he does is open his overnight bag.

264

From it he takes a large envelope. He extracts from it what looks like a certificate. And with his face completely dead-pan he hands it to his father.

Colin's jaw drops. Then his face breaks into an enormous grin.

"Well done, son!" He jumps up to shake Andrew's hand as I grab the piece of paper.

This is to certify

that Andrew Belshaw who attended Private Pilot Licence course number 012 at 43 Air School, Port Alfred from 8 January 1990 to 28 January 1990 was adjudged by the panel of Flying Instructors and the Flight Safety Officer to be the pilot whose actions, both on the ground and in the air, demonstrated the highest standard of Airmanship.

- 0 -

The leg was deteriorating rapidly. It was enormously swollen and discoloured and looked absolutely ghastly.

"How on earth did you fly at all with your leg like this," I asked Andrew.

He grinned that wicked grin of his. "Easy. I put a pressure pad on it and just kept it in a tight tuby-grip the whole time."

"What about the pain."

"I told the pain to go away. Like you told me to."

I smiled. "How it didn't burst during one of your training flights I'll never understand. It's a miracle it waited until you were back in Manchester."

Thinking about it that night I realised that the real miracle was that everything happened because Andrew had made it happen. It was his goal to be a pilot. It was his determination, and it was his sheer will power in keeping the leg intact, that had made him succeed.

On Thursday we packed our suitcases and at four-thirty on Friday morning we drove up to London, with Andrew stretched out on the back seat.

Sister O'Leary, who had been in charge of the orthopaedic surgery wards five years ago, ruling with her rod of iron, was still there, and

265

she and Andrew greeted each other like old friends. Grey haired now, she seemed to have softened and mellowed. We were able to get to know her better this time because of the new flexible visiting hours, and found that beneath that super-efficient mask lay understanding and empathy which for some reason I had not perceived before. She put Andrew in a single ward with two large windows, a bathroom-en-suite and a remote controlled television set. Wow! What luxury!

Mr Sweetnam and his team were at first uncertain of their plan of action. "We will open up the leg again and see what is happening, and why. We may find it necessary to replace the existing prosthesis with a new one," he said. "Or we might patch up everything with new cement."

The third option was left unspoken.

The operation was scheduled for the following Thursday and all Andrew could think of was getting it over with so that he could start flying again and get his PPL.

On Wednesday night he seemed quieter than usual.

"Are you okay, Andrew?" I asked. "Have you signed the consent form yet?"

He nodded. "I signed it."

Then he smiled a little half smile. "There's no point in making a big fuss, like I used to do. If they have to do what they have to do, then that's okay with me. I signed for everything."

I knew what that meant. I felt the familiar icy cold shudder down my spine.

On Thursday afternoon we crept in quietly. He was surrounded by drips and tubes and a big cage over his leg. Turning back the clock I peeped under the cover.

I have counted your toes ...

And there are ten!

This time the pain was being very effectively controlled by a drip administering the pain-killing drug, which unfortunately had to be stopped after two days because it caused nausea and vomiting.

Visiting hours were free and easy now. Philip and Jo popped in regularly and so did all Andrew's friends. The atmosphere in the ward was relaxed and cheerful, the efficiency as high as ever.

We asked Mr Sweetnam what they had done this time, and what the black patches in the swollen area were.

"We cleared away all the granulation tissue and the fluid," he

266

explained, "and we hope that by filling the cavity in the bone with a special new antibiotic cement, we may be able to stop the reaction, and stop the titanium leaching into the surrounding tissues which we think could be causing the inflammation. We did think we might have needed to replace the prosthesis," he went on, "but in fact we found there'd been no loosening or mechanical failure, which are the more likely problems with these replacements."

"Does that mean everything will be fine now," I asked.

"We can't promise. It'll be a few days before we get the lab reports but we don't think there's any deep-seated infection there. We don't know why the bone has deteriorated. Or what's causing the reaction between the bone and the metal. It may well settle down. We'll just have to wait and see."

He directed his gaze at Andrew. "But he'll have to be very careful from now on. No high jinks, and he must remain on crutches for two months after the stitches have been removed."

A look of horror descended on Andrew's face. "Oh! Does that mean no flying?"

"No work. No driving. No swimming. No scuba diving. No more walking than is absolutely necessary. And *definitely* no flying, Andrew. For at *least* two months."

On the tenth day the stitches came out and the results from the lab were all negative. Two days later Andrew was discharged and we took him home to Wilmslow.

- 0 -

It was a long two months and difficult for Andrew to come to terms with the almost total immobility. His biggest weapon against his illness and the problems with his leg had always been his very positive attitude, and this time he used every power which he believed would hasten the healing and reduce the pain: Positive thinking. Relaxation. Visualisation. Language behaviour. Large doses of Vitamin C – no less than one thousand milligrams a day.

And sheer determination.

Every day the sounds of the cello filled the house. So intense, so moving, so poignant was the emotion in his playing that at times I could almost feel his pain being released through the passion he poured out through the instrument. I also felt that in some intrinsic

267

way he was communicating with the resonating notes, imploring them to come back into his body to hasten the healing process.

At last it was time for the final check-up at The Middlesex. He was given the all-clear to go back to work. Singapore Airlines had waited patiently for his return and welcomed him back with open arms. The manager, Jim Belch, who I so often over the years could have hugged for taking Andrew on in the first place, and still would like to do if given the chance, never failed to demonstrate his unusually humane qualities of understanding and compassion.

Colin went back to Menorca to see to problems we were having with our house. I decided to stay with Andrew a little longer until I was certain he no longer needed my help.

- 0 -

At last the crutches were abandoned. He was down to using only one stick and was thrilled to be back into the swing at work.

- 0 -

A few days later he phones me from the office and tells me he will be home a couple of hours later than usual.

"Oh. Where are you going?" I ask inquisitively, hoping it might be a new girlfriend. He is so full of love. He needs someone to share his life with and pour out his love to, but since Julie he has found no-one yet who has the sensitivity or the understanding or the gentleness to take her place.

"Flying," he says.

My heart lurches.

Flying? But what if the operation has made his leg even weaker? And what if he doesn't have the strength to work the rudder pedals?

Then I get a grip on myself.

Damn it! He's going to do what he always wanted to do, I remind myself firmly. For him there can be no greater happiness.

All afternoon I pace up and down the house. I drink cups of Rooibos tea. I gaze out of the window. I play Beethoven's Emperor Concerto over and over again, tears rolling down my cheeks in the slow second movement – the most beautiful adagio ever written. At last I see the car in the driveway and rush to the front door.

268

I watch him get out of the car. See him turn the key in the lock. Now he is walking towards me ...

He smiles.

Never before have I seen a face so filled with joy.

"I've been flying, Mum."

- 0 -

Whenever we were back in Wilmslow it was always Andrew's future agenda that was the main topic of conversation. Quite clearly he was not content just to hold a PPL.

"I don't care how long it takes me, Dad. But I must get a Commercial Pilot Licence. Five years. Ten years. I'm going to do it. I must."

Colin saw the grit and determination reflected in the firm set of Andrew's mouth. He understood his son's all-consuming ambition but could see a multitude of stumbling blocks standing in his way. As a young man he had had the same ravenous need and he couldn't bear the thought of Andrew also not realising his dreams. It would not be easy to make him change his mind, yet he had to try.

"Your leg could be a problem, Andrew. Without a Class 1 medical certificate you would be restricted – you probably wouldn't be allowed to fly passengers. The training is very time consuming. Very difficult. And very, very expensive. You've already used up all your money getting your PPL, but Commercial Pilot training is a different story. It costs far more than you've got."

"I'll find the money somehow, Dad. I'll carry on working at Singapore Airlines and in my spare time I can make quite a bit working part-time in the control tower at Barton."

Barton was in Eccles, in north Manchester. It had been Manchester's first civil airport, long before Ringway (later Manchester Airport) was built. It was now the home of the Lancashire Aero Club which Andrew had joined when he'd decided to complete his PPL in England. They were always looking for regular people to operate the radio in the control tower.

It was also where later he would meet Sally.

After Mr Sweetnam had given him the all-clear to start flying again, he had lived and breathed flying and had soon got his UK PPL; but the Commercial Pilot Licence was his new dream.

269

In Andrew's eyes there was only one snag.

Right now he had only one hundred and four flying hours under his belt. To get your CPL you had to have two hundred. This would be horrendously expensive to achieve.

Colin looked at his son. He saw the longing in his eyes. Remembered how the world had ended when his own father had stopped him taking up his place at RAF College, Cranwell.

And he made a decision: *Give him the flowers now.*

"You could do it in South Africa," he said. "It'll be far cheaper there."

Andrew frowned. "I know, Dad, but I can't afford to give up my job at Singapore Airlines. I need the money. Besides, I can't stay out of England for long because of my leg check-ups."

"Once you've passed the written exams and clocked up a good few hours in South Africa, you could come back to England and get a job while you continue to notch up your hours here. Singapore Airlines might even take you back!"

Andrew looked at his father with awe-struck eyes as slowly the penny dropped. *His father was offering to sponsor him.*

Very sadly he resigned from Singapore Airlines who had been so good to him, and in October 1991, beside himself with excitement, he went back to 43 Air school.

- 0 -

He stayed in South Africa for six months, but before leaving he did something incredible.

Something that TS Eliot would have agreed made it all worth while. Even compensating for his disappointment at 43 Air School.

Something that ascended beyond the outer reaches of his dreams.

Chapter Twenty-eight

1992

Dear Dad,

You wanted a blow-by-blow description of my adventure, so here it is.

It all started as a joke really. I said to Trevor – he was my best mate at 43 Air School – 'Let's fly to Lusaka after the exams.' Okay, I know. Nearly two thousand miles there and two thousand miles back – depending on our route. A bit daft but it seemed like a good idea. A once in a lifetime experience I never thought could happen.

Trevor and I had struck up a firm friendship. As the end of the course approached we were desperate for a change of scenery, even though Port Alfred was incredibly beautiful with wide open beaches stretching for miles both east and west. But it wasn't the bit of Africa I really wanted to see. I really wanted to go 'home'.

I arranged to meet Trev in Pietermaritzburg a few days after the exams ended. I'd planned to hire a Cherokee 140 from Pro Aviation in George, fly east to Port Elizabeth and onwards for what I hoped would be a non-stop trouble-free flight to Kwa-Zulu Natal. I would collect Trevor there and we would then fly together up to Lanseria Airport in Jo'burg on the first leg of our journey north.

271

We hadn't received our results yet. I was a bit worried about this and was not confident about passing. I'd felt pretty lousy during the exams, along with others who'd also had that awful debilitating bug.

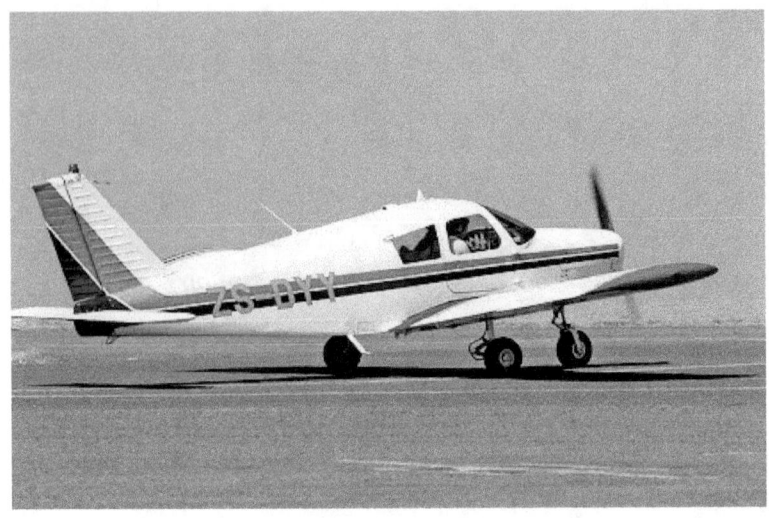

The Cherokee 140 – ZS-DYY that Andrew and Trevor flew from George to Lusaka and back

The day I was due to leave George, the Cherokee 140 – Zulu Sierra Delta Yankee Yankee (ZS-DYY) – had a magneto drop. I was then delayed a further day because of bad weather but eventually got away on my first really long flight on my tod. I landed as planned at Port Elizabeth, refuelled and set off for Pietermaritzburg.

I'd just passed East London when I hit bad weather. The cloud base was getting lower and lower. I thought about trying to punch my way through but I was already down to about three hundred feet above the waves. On a sunny day it would have been exhilarating but in this wild weather it was not a lot of fun.

Can't say I was very happy, and wondered if I should battle on or turn back. I decided that discretion would be

272

the better part of valour and banked through one hundred and eighty degrees and set course for East London.

The weather got worse. I was shit scared. What was I doing flying in these foul conditions? I had to get to East London before it got any worse.

After several frightening minutes I finally saw the airfield. I was the only thing still flying. Even the birds were on the ground.

At last I was established on final approach and had the runway lights gleaming ahead of me. There was thick low cloud and a gusty wind across the runway. The landing was not so pretty on this occasion!

I know what you're saying, Dad. And you're right. But in spite of what you might call my stupidity in being in that weather at all, it felt like the best landing I had ever made, as there was no way I could have gone around again into that still lowering cloud base.

You once reminded me – remember? – 'There are old pilots and bold pilots, but no old bold pilots.'

I learned a lesson about flying in bad weather that day! What a fool I'd been to even try such an idiotic thing. I should have landed at East London in the first place.

Anyway, the following morning I took off into a perfect blue sky. My three hour flight to Pietermaritzburg took me over a stunningly clear and beautiful coastline as far as Port St Johns, then inland across totally unfamiliar countryside – miles and miles of pale brown bushland and rolling hills with now and then a small patch of green where a river wound its way down towards the sea.

273

Trev was waiting on the tarmac. We quickly refuelled, filed our flight plans, checked all was in order and departed for Jo'burg. It was the time of the year when thunderstorms are common in the late afternoon and early evening, and we had to fly around massive storm clouds stretching up as high as 50,000 feet. I could hear your voice telling me, 'Don't fly anywhere near a thunderstorm!' Yeah, don't tell me – little aeroplanes and cumulonimbus clouds don't mix.

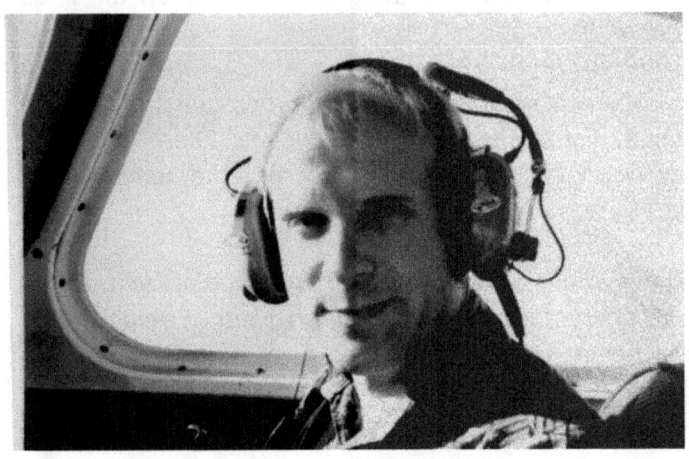

On our way to Zambia

During the last phase of our three hour journey to Lanseria the sun set in a blaze of orange and pink, and we flew the final hour at night. Spectacular displays of lightning like the fiesta fireworks in Menorca lit up the night sky all around us. They seemed so near but were actually miles away from DYY. I must say it was an interesting experience flying at night in such busy unfamiliar airspace. Silly really to have attempted it at all but I had a night rating and I was jolly well going to use it.

We spent the next morning acquiring a hand-held radio and attempting to fix the VOR. We also organised a GPS, a great piece of satellite navigation kit that you didn't have in the days when you were flying. It was a godsend and worked perfectly the whole way to Zambia and back.

We left at mid-day and flew a direct route to Bulawayo. This was a nostalgic part of the journey for me. It was strange to think I'd been at boarding school there from the age of six to eleven. I hadn't been back since, and was surprised to see how small the city had grown!

After landing we refuelled and filed for a direct track to Kariba, but believe it or not, until we were airborne we didn't know that Kariba airport was due to close before we were due to land! This was bad news, Dad, because without refuelling at Kariba we hadn't a hope of continuing on to Lusaka.

Bulawayo Air Traffic Control came to the rescue. They were great. They contacted Kariba and persuaded them to stay open. We landed two hours later after a breathtaking descent over the lake, approaching straight into a burning sunset which bathed the surface of the water in a furnace of reds and orange. Okay, I know that sounds corny, but it really was like nothing I'd ever seen before.

Our departure from Kariba was equally spectacular. We had just become airborne when a herd of about fifty elephants on their evening stroll began approaching the opposite end of the runway. We flew low over their heads, as they do in wildlife films and I wished I'd had my camera handy. They seemed totally untroubled by us but we were spellbound.

The final stage of the journey was entirely at night. One hour and twenty minutes of peaceful flying through the African sky. All we could hear was the drone of the engine as Trevor and I sat in silence with our thoughts, not really sure if it was a dream or reality as we drew nearer to our final destination – Lusaka.

Such a strange exciting feeling to be landing this little aeroplane in the country where I was born!

There were few lights on the ground and our radio navigation aids were unreliable, so it was useful to have a lot of local knowledge. Finally we could see the runway lights at Lusaka International. Out there in the middle of the bush they were unmistakable, as I'm sure you'll remember. I was so excited as we touched down, realising that finally the dream had come true.

We were collected by an old friend of mine and driven off down the familiar airport road. It was like I'd never been away, Dad. We wound our way through Chainama and Kalingalinga, past the golf club where I'd played as a teenager and the Olympic size pool where I'd played water polo every Wednesday. It was wonderful to be back on familiar turf, and sad when after two magical days we had to go back to Lusaka International to begin our long journey back to the Cape.

You wouldn't believe it. Before we could leave, the guy in the tower insisted that we complete several forms in triplicate. Where we were from and where we were going and all that stuff. Control finally gave us our clearance and thanks to my local knowledge and our sat nav aid, we were able to carry out our intricate instructions – you'd have thought we were a Boeing 747! – this time heading to one of my favourite places on earth, where we used to go when I was just a kid. Livingstone, and the fantastic Vic Falls.

After a two and a half hour flight we saw the spray. You can see it exploding into the sky from miles around. We called up Livingstone on the radio and they gave us joining instructions to land. It was disappointing not to overfly the Falls on our approach but we could do that

276

the following day.

We spent the night at Rainbow Lodge on the banks of the Zambezi. From the restaurant there's a stunning rainbow view of the spray, and even after all the times I'd seen it before it was still magnificent. The noise is so deafening that it's no wonder the local people call it Mosi o Tunya – the smoke that thunders.

As the sun went down and the chatter of monkeys subsided, the bush came alive with the chirping of crickets and that whistling noise the little green tree-frogs make, and the grunts of hippos munching away on the river banks. And all the time the continuous thunder from the torrents of water plunging over the Falls. It's a symphony of sound you can only hear in Africa.

Next morning we were back at Livingstone airport for our short hop across the border from Zambia to Zim. We loaded our bags, did our walk round, then taxied out and took off for Vic Falls airport.

I could never have believed it would be so fantastic. Doing steep turns first one way and then the other, we spent an exhilarating half an hour flying around the Falls. It looks quite different from the air. You must do it some time, Dad. The river, from being a sedate flow of dark greys and browns suddenly becomes a rage of turbulent whites and greens and yellows as it disappears over the edge and tumbles down the rock face into the depths below. The spray is so dense that it's sometimes impossible to see into the gorge. Then suddenly the river takes on its original sedate form.

Eventually we dragged ourselves away and set course for Vic Falls airport. Where once more, disaster almost struck.

Despite a thorough pre-flight inspection before we left

Livingstone, the right undercarriage oleo had obviously developed some sort of fault. I had visions of making a landing on one wheel. Of the wing hitting ground. Of the runway ripping into the now extended flaps. How were we going to explain away a broken aeroplane to the guys in George?

We struggled to keep her straight and it was only through luck rather than judgement that we stayed on the runway.

I'm glad my metal leg worked. If it hadn't we would have been in bad trouble.

With a jolt we stopped. The undercarriage was still there although the oleo had lost all the hydraulic compression available. How we would get out of this mess we did not know. We taxied with extreme care and as we parked up, we noticed a South African Airways Airbus on the ground. After much waving at the crew, who were amused to see a little old aeroplane so far from home, their engineer came over to us and offered his assistance. He also managed to persuade the Zimbabwe ground crew to help, and they did a temporary repair job so we could continue our journey. After much laughing and joking with our benefactors (this SAA crew thought we were mad flying such a long way in our little machine – "Man, you guys are only crazy, hey!") we took off on the longest stretch of our journey: nearly four hours flying to Messina.

What a flight! You'd have loved it, Dad. Our route took us over the Hwange National Game Reserve where you and Mum often took me on the way home from school in Bulawayo up to the Copperbelt. It was teeming with game, but we were shocked to see how badly the countryside had been devastated by the severe drought. You just wouldn't recognise it. And when we got to the Zim-SA border near Messina, an even more amazing *sight was the Limpopo River. Almost completely dry!*

The rest of the journey, between Messina and Newcastle and onwards to Pietermaritzburg, was no less fascinating. What sunsets! I always tell my friends there's nothing more stunning than an African sunset, but from the air the colours seem even more vivid and more widely splashed.

We had more thunderstorms to dodge. And more night flying too, so smooth without the heat from the sun causing updrafts from the surface that tended to toss our little machine around like a toy. Which I'm sure you remember well from your days of flying at Kitwe and Williamson Diamonds. It was a good thing I'd become qualified to fly at night. I wouldn't have missed it for anything.

I left Trevor in Pietermaritzburg and flew on to Margate where he met me later. We spent a week there, swimming and sunbathing and generally taking it easy. I went to visit the Armstrongs, just a few miles down the Natal coast. Hadn't seen them since I was a kid in Zambia and it was strange to see familiar things in their house. Like the model planes you gave them so many years ago, Dad, when you used to spend hours building models.

We flew the now familiar route back to base, along the coast to East London, then to Plett Bay, and finally to George.

All in all we'd spent about forty hours inside that little Cherokee 140. It was almost as though she became part of us. We could recognise every sound she made and it was a sad moment to have to say goodbye to her.

It was the end of an adventure. An almost 4000 mile journey across Africa we never really thought was possible and yet we had done it. Although we'd been in a fairly modern aeroplane, I could now imagine what it must have been like back in the early days of aviation, battling with the elements in open cockpits and planes built of wood. But they did it, and only now could I appreciate their difficulties.

My leg had been brilliant. I had some discomfort – it was a long way to sit in a little plane. But what a way to see Africa!

And what a way to fulfil a dream.

Thanks a million, Dad.

All my love,

Andrew

Chapter Twenty-nine

1992 – 1995

Andrew arrived back in England in April 1992. He had no money left and it looked as though he must abandon his ambition. Alas, he had not passed the CPL written exams because as luck would have it, just before the candidates were flown to Port Elizabeth for the examinations, Andrew, together with one or two other pilots, caught a bad dose of the virulent flu that was doing the rounds. He soldiered on, but during most of the exams he had a high temperature and ended up with five points less than the required pass mark.

While trying to decide what to do next he accepted the offer of a regular position at Barton Aerodrome, operating the radio in the control tower.

Being on the spot, he also took every opportunity to fly.

- 0 -

One Saturday afternoon in May he was on duty in the tower. It was a clear, sunny day, though windy. To the north he could see Winter Hill. To the east Barton Bridge – the big high-level bridge over the Manchester Ship Canal – and to the south the city. One of the many things Andrew loved about working in the tower was the vista of miles of sky stretching beyond the unknown limits of sight that had so intrigued him in Africa. Down below, parked to the left and the right of the tower, were rows of light aircraft. Well over a hundred little aeroplanes that he would drool over and dream of one day flying beyond those unknown limits, just as he and Trevor had done in South and Central Africa.

The airfield was buzzing with activity. The sky was full of the drone of small aircraft, and every few minutes planes were either taking off or landing.

He was busy working the radio when a pretty, vivacious girl came

281

up the stairs to talk to a friend of hers who was also helping out in the tower.

She didn't seem to notice Andrew, although she did say hello.

But Andrew certainly noticed her.

He noticed first her lively blue eyes, her radiant smile, and then her shapely figure, especially her legs and her incredibly slim ankles. She was wearing a black and white checked skirt, red shoes that matched her red blouse, and a black jacket with a gold road-runner brooch on the lapel.

He'd been just about to say something to her when he was forced to drag his eyes away to talk to two planes approaching the landing strip. They both landed safely, but by the time they had taxied in over the uneven grass, the girl had gone.

Ten minutes later there was a lull in the movements so he idly looked down from the tower to see what was going on around the hangars.

His luck was in. There she was! Standing talking animatedly to someone near the flat-topped building that was the clubhouse.

His heart skipped a beat. She was so alive looking, so vital; and even from the tower he could see the alert, intelligent look on her face.

The south west wind swept her red silk blouse against the slim curves of her body and blew her blonde hair across her eyes.

Andrew was totally captivated.

So much so that at first he had hardly noticed that holding her hands were two little girls.

"Just my luck," he muttered under his breath.

He sighed, and concentrated on the sky around him.

Then one day in August everything changed.

He entered for the annual Landing Competition, competing for the coveted Rodman Trophy – a large silver cup on which many illustrious names in the world of aviation were engraved.

"What is this Landing Competition," I asked. "I hope it's not too dangerous."

Andrew laughed. "It's quite easy, Mum. Each pilot takes off and climbs to overhead the airfield, chops the engine and then has to perform a glide approach to the runway, landing over a rope suspended across the runway threshold, as close as possible to the rope."

"With no engine!" I said, horrified.

282

"It's good practice for when you have an engine failure," Andrew explained. "The pilot is judged not only on landing nearest the rope but by the accuracy of the flying, the neatness of the circuit, as well as the standard of the landing."

The weather was scorching. There were over fifty entries. At the end of the day everyone gathered in the clubhouse. Whose name, they all wondered, would be the next one to be engraved on the big silver trophy.

As they waited for the announcement the excitement was electric.

The names were read out. There was only one point between Andrew and the pretty blonde girl.

Andrew had won! He had beaten the pretty blonde girl into second place.

Her name was Sally.

Sally was also very ambitious. As one of the best pilots in the club she was unhappy with second place. She asked her friend:

"Who is this Andy Belshaw?"

Although she had said hello to him in the tower she had never been introduced, so did not associate the name with the person she'd seen that day. When she was told she said, incredulously, "You mean that guy with the gammy leg in the tower is the guy who beat me?"

The prize-giving was at the annual Wings Dinner Dance in November. It was a scintillating occasion, held at the Valley Lodge Hotel in Wilmslow. There was a live band. Everyone was dressed to kill.

Andrew found himself scanning the sea of lively faces for one face in particular. Nowhere could he see her. Surely she would be here, he thought, his hopes beginning to fade.

And then he saw her, looking stunning in a shimmering blue ball gown.

He couldn't take his eyes off her, but although he kept looking in her direction he could not catch her eye.

Years later Sally told me she could see him looking at her. Out of the corner of her eye she was looking at him too. She couldn't quite make him out. She wondered what it was about him that seemed so appealing. Although he laughed a lot and seemed a very warm kind of person, there was a certain ... she didn't know quite what it was ... almost a kind of melancholy ... a sad, thoughtful pensiveness that she perceived in spite of the jovial exterior. She wondered too why underneath his eyes there were such dark rings.

She felt herself becoming more and more curious. She wanted to get to know him. It was a very formal occasion but although he appeared not to have brought anyone with him, she decided to keep her distance.

Andrew's name was called. He grasped his stick and walked to the top table to receive his Bronze Wings. Sally noted the look of serene pleasure on his face.

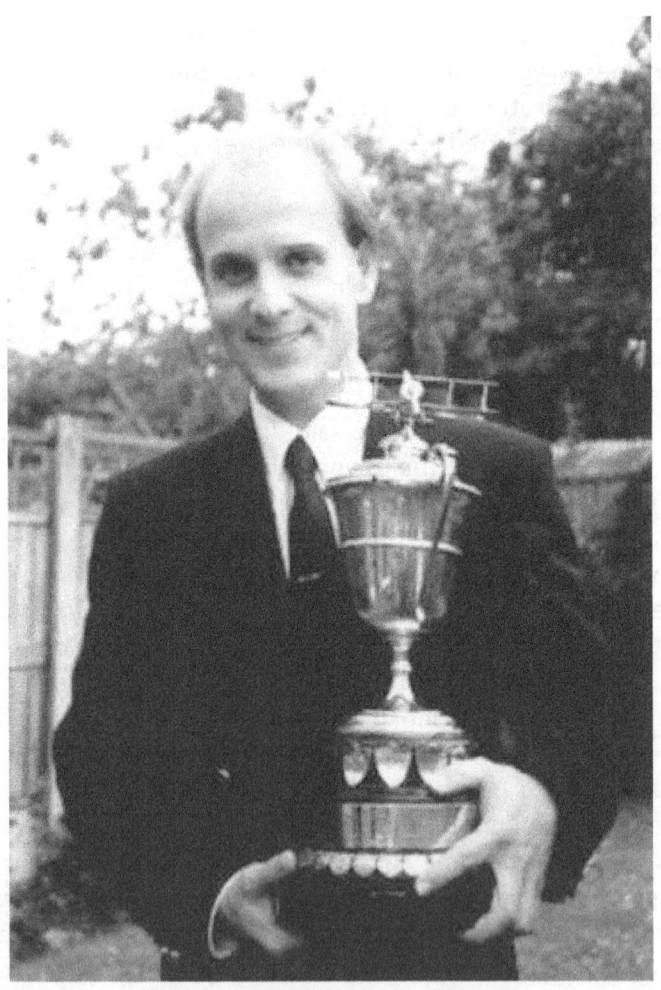

Andrew with Rodman Trophy

At last it was time for the presentation of the Rodman Trophy. The winner's name was announced. To thunderous applause Andrew stood up, so elated that this time he didn't even think of taking his stick. Walking on air he reached the top table. Amid the deafening applause he collected his gleaming trophy. To get back to his seat he had to walk right past Sally.

Just as he passed her she looked straight into his eyes.

He stopped dead in his tracks and stared back at her, suddenly flustered when she held out her hand and said, "Congratulations, Andrew Belshaw."

"Thank you," he said, quite taken aback.

"But I am not amused," Sally said with a smile on her face and a twinkle in her eyes that nearly knocked Andrew over. "Next year I'll take that trophy off you!"

Andrew loved a challenge, but he was also a gentleman. He smiled.

"It will be my pleasure," he said, and floated back to his seat.

Later in the evening, when everything became less formal, Sally approached his table. The white silk scarf that adorned his black dinner suit hung loose around his neck. Playfully she took hold of the ends and tried to pull him up.

"Come and dance, Andrew."

"I can't," Andrew said, seized with unaccustomed shyness. "My leg _"

"I'll be gentle," Sally said. She took off his scarf and draped it round her own neck.

- 0 -

Soon afterwards, on a cold wet blustery overcast afternoon when no-one was mad enough to fly their aircraft, Andrew wandered down from the tower for a cup of coffee in the clubhouse.

He stopped breathing. There she was. Her back was to him but her two daughters looked up as he came through the door.

"Hi," he said, not quite sure what else to say to such little girls.

Sally turned round. "Oh, Hi," she said. "Want a coffee?"

"I'll get them," Andrew said. "What would the girls like?"

When he came back to the table Sally introduced her daughters. The eldest, Rebecca, and little Alex, only three. Both had long dark silky hair and large brown eyes. They looked up at Andrew and then quickly down at their feet, their dark lashes curling across their pearl white cheeks.

After that they often bumped into each other at the clubhouse, and found they had a great deal in common.

They had both always wanted to fly. They both had Private Pilot Licences. They both wanted to become Commercial Pilots.

Her children adored him. They quickly became really good friends and started throwing ideas around about seriously becoming commercial pilots – about where, when and how to do it. Even though there was no chance of any grant or sponsorship, Andrew decided to resume his training as and when funds permitted, and Sally also started her training.

Their joint goal cemented their friendship. Yet it was only when she invited him to a New Year's party at her house, that love blossomed.

- 0 -

Financially the training was an uphill struggle. For both of them to achieve their goal they were looking at a sum of money way beyond their means, or even their capacity to borrow.

And Sally it was who helped Andrew with his heart-breaking decision.

"You're wasting your money, Andy. With your leg you'll never be an airline pilot. Even though you've now managed to get a Class 2 Flying Medical it'll never enable you to carry passengers. You could become a flying instructor but that hardly pays a living wage."

Andrew listened to her without saying a word. He knew that everything she was saying was true. He had known it all along but his burning desire to be a Commercial Pilot had blotted out all reason.

"For me too," Sally said wistfully. "I just can't carry on. I'm a single mother now. Two small children. The cost is crippling me. Even if I do make it, I can't leave the children for days on end."

"What are you saying, Sally?" His eyes misted up. "That we must both give up our dreams?"

They sat looking at each other across the table. She took his hand. Her dreams were evaporating too but she had made up her mind that one of them had to face realities and it was obvious it would have to be her.

"We could become air traffic controllers instead," she said softly.

Andrew slowly shook his head. He gazed into her eyes and saw that she meant it.

"And stop *flying*?"

"We'd still be closely connected to flying. Our experience would stand us in good stead. We'd understand the problems."

"Yes, we would." Andrew's voice was so low it was barely audible.

"The pay is good. You said you wanted to be a controller once. It was only your leg that made the RAF reject you. You love your work in the Barton tower. Think how much more satisfying it would be to work in a real tower."

Andrew's lifelong dream – his lifelong ambition – was slipping away but he knew Sally was right.

"Okay," he said, pulling himself together as he always does. "I've been giving ATC a lot of thought myself," he admitted. "Let's make enquiries about training. It'll be a challenge."

They were on their own. Sponsorship was not an option. Taking a giant step, they borrowed a vast amount of money from the bank and took themselves off to the Aviation Foundation Training Centre in Bournemouth.

It would be sink –

Or swim.

A few weeks later Andrew bought Sally a ring and they became engaged. The following year they both qualified as Air Traffic Control Officers. It was an arduous course, formidable and gruelling, but they succeeded.

- 0 -

In October, twelve months after they become engaged, Colin and I flew over from Menorca for the wedding. It was a happy occasion – for me especially, for I had been afraid he would remain so wrapped up in his flying that he would never leave room for a family life. Or for the love he was so capable of giving.

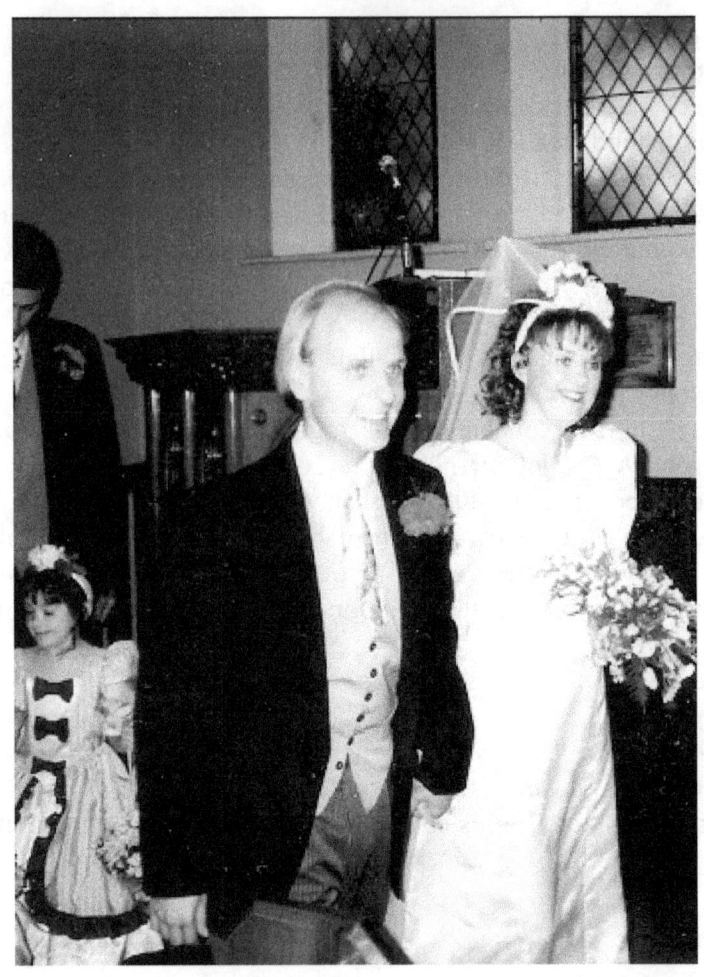

Andrew & Sally's wedding at Hartford Hall, Cheshire in October 1994

Sally looked radiant in her long, full dress of ivory shantung, and Andrew, now the father of two lovely little dark haired girls, was in seventh heaven. His old school friend, Cor Roest, was best man, and Stuart an usher. Peter and Andrea were there with their children, Katie and Matthew, and so were the Baverstocks, but we sorely missed our eldest son Colin, and Philip and Jo, who were unable to come.

After the speeches the music started. Smiling that big smile of his, Andrew led his bride onto the floor. I watched him dance. I was all choked up, suddenly remembering his gallant effort at Peter's wedding when he'd insisted on going once around the floor.

As they stood at the door of the church and the confetti flew through the air I felt a warm surge of love and relief and satisfaction all rolled into one. How strange that happiness at a wedding should bring forth tears.

- 0 -

The following day, in the void one is left with after an event of intense emotion, I marvelled that throughout all the excitement Andrew had not once complained about his leg.

Chapter Thirty

1995 – 1997

Andrew's first job as a qualified Air Traffic Controller was at Netheravon Army Base in Wiltshire. From the moment he started he loved it. In his spare time he shot small bore rifle for Wiltshire, and devoted three evenings a week helping to run a local detached flight in the RAF Air Training Corps. On his days off he drove home to be with Sally and the girls.

His life seemed at last to be perfect. Except for one thing.

His leg was constantly painful.

It was swollen again and the skin badly stained by the titanium leaching into the tissues. Every day it had to be bandaged and encased in a full length elastic stocking. Eventually the inevitable happened, as it did in 1990 when he arrived back from South Africa.

> *The leg burst open.*
> *Oozing*
> *Blue black gunge*
> *Clear yellow fluid.*
> *Not too painful now, but I know I have a problem*
> *Just at the wrong time*
> *Sally starting her new job tomorrow.*

Sally rushed him to the local Accident and Emergency. As before, the only course of action was an operation at The Middlesex.

> *Back in The Middlesex*
> *Bond Street Ward.*
> *Mr Cobb and his team*
> *Green masks. Knives.*
> *Everything fine*
> *Till the pain control machine runs out.*

Pain builds up.
Nurses busy. Not time yet for their drugs round.
I can bear it no longer, then suddenly
Framed in the doorway
Like an angel
Sally appears

What can she think?
Me
Behaving like an idiot.
Crying like a child
Writhing on the bed
In agony.

Something for the pain, please, she says.
Not later when you're ready
But now.
A nurse hurries to my bedside
Apologising,
Clutching a handful of pills.

Sally. Sitting on my bed. Holding my hand.
Are you thirsty? Hungry? Is there anything I can do?
Still muzzy from the morphine I nod.
Sally. Spoon feeds me. Peaches
Like Nectar
But they all come back.

She smiles.
Cleans me up
Strokes my brow
Holds my hand
Smiles again
Like an angel

- 0 -

That year was not a good one for Andrew's leg. Five months after that operation, arriving one morning for physiotherapy at Salisbury Hospital, ten miles from Netheravon, Andrew slipped on wet grass while taking a short-cut to the entrance.

The agony of the fall made him scream with pain. He was filled with horror and fear that the leg might be broken and have to be amputated. By the time he got back to Netheravon from the hospital the pain was unbearable. Every time he moved, bone rubbed against metal. He couldn't sleep. He couldn't even walk or stand or sit because every movement caused excruciating pain.

He was rushed to The Middlesex.

Andrew was no longer being treated by Sir Rodney Sweetnam who was now retired, although he held the position of Emeritus Head of the Department of Orthopaedic Surgery at The Middlesex as well as President of the Royal College of Surgeons. His successor, Mr Justin Cobb, who'd been treating Andrew since 1991, found that the prosthesis had loosened again and operated immediately.

Once again Mr Cobb patched up the leg as best he could, re-cementing the prosthesis into the crumbling bone. The day after the operation he visited Andrew.

"I must warn you, Andrew, that the time is fast approaching when vital decisions will have to be made. The prosthesis is becoming old and worn. It will have to be replaced."

Andrew lay back on his pillows, still groggy from the anaesthetic.

"I've been expecting you to say that for ages, Mr Cobb. When do you think you'll do it?"

Mr Cobb pondered this for a moment. "It's not so much when we'll do it, but if the leg will stand up to this treatment."

Andrew had great confidence in Mr Cobb. "He always tells me the facts, Mum. Though not always what I want to hear. We're able to speak freely to each other and that's what I really like."

Mr Cobb is a tall, slim man whose unbounded energy is exceeded only by his dedication to his profession. Softly spoken and down to earth, he is always encouraging, but never fudges what it is necessary to say.

"We could make a new prosthesis now," he told Andrew. "We could open up the leg. But the grave danger lies in the possibility that we might find that the small amount of remaining tibia which has been eroding away all these years, is not strong enough to withstand the fitting of a new prosthesis."

292

Andrew looked long and hard at his surgeon.

"What then, Mr Cobb?"

"We would have to amputate the leg."

- 0 -

The Middlesex Hospital's new 'Pain Team' had been progressively improving their management of pain control, so Andrew's latest repair operation was easier to tolerate than in previous years, and within six weeks he was back in the tower at Netheravon.

A few weeks later there was much rejoicing when he was commissioned as a Pilot Officer in the RAF Volunteer Reserve, Training Branch. He phoned us with the news.

"And guess what, Dad."

"I know!" replied his father, brimful with pride. And, I suspect, a little bit of nostalgic jealousy. "You have a blue uniform to go with it. And a blue flat hat!"

"At last! I can't believe it. Me! In the RAF!"

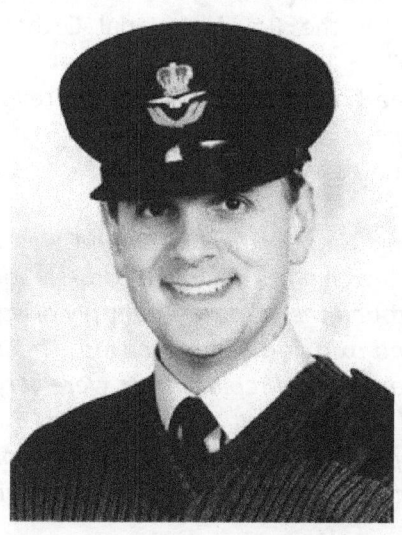

Excited to be wearing the RAF Reserve Uniform

- 0 -

The leg continued to give trouble.

Mr Cobb discussed a possible replacement with Andrew and finally decided they could no longer delay. On his thirty-first birthday in September 1996 Andrew was admitted to The Middlesex for his eighth operation.

We were five thousand miles away in Zambia where Colin was doing a three-year post-retirement contract at the request of the World Bank, helping the copper mining industry to get back on its feet.

As usual there was the threat of amputation and I would have given anything to be there in London with Andrew. But he had Sally now and I didn't think it would be appropriate for me to be hovering around as well. We had the usual sleepless night worrying about whether he would lose his leg or not.

But this time it was different.

So different that it took us completely by surprise.

Mr Cobb rebuilt the leg.

Not just with a new prosthesis but with a new, revolutionary experimental prosthesis funded by the Medical Research Council, which he and Dr Gordon Blunn had been researching at the Biomedical Engineering Centre at the Royal National Orthopaedic Hospital in Stanmore since 1992.

We'd had no idea how much research and revolutionary progress had been taking place.

In his operation notes Mr Cobb wrote:

After preparing the leg the old wound was re-opened along its entire length and the grossly discoloured membrane around the prosthesis sharply dissected after the bushes and axle had been removed. The lugs of the titanium proximal tibial replacement were very seriously worn and the axle itself was damaged. The distal femoral component was made of cast cobalt chrome and seemed to be very firmly fixed and so this was not removed.

The distal tibial bone was resected as planned at 24mm in the transaction plane, and after shaping the bone ends the extra-cortical plate fixation was hammered

294

into place. The procedure itself went extremely well but I couldn't quite ground the prosthesis. The anterolateral and anteromedial plates were further fixed with screws. After this there was no trace of movement possible with twisting or bending or of course pulling or pushing.

After lavage with 1500 mls of saline the wound was closed with Vicryl to layers and skin, but considerable undercutting was necessary to ensure the layers were closed without tension.

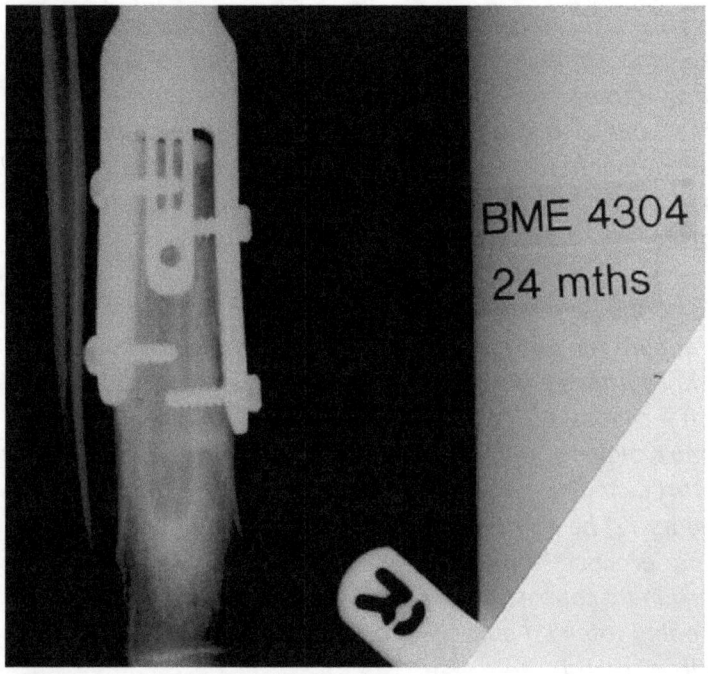

New prosthesis, 24 months later

So what was the vital difference in layman's terms?

Andrew faxed us a sketch which he did from an X-ray of the new titanium prosthesis which showed that the vital difference between the old intra-medullary cemented stem prosthesis and the new one, was that the old one fitted into the bone, whereas the new one fitted over and around the bone with its three extra-cortical plates screwed

295

into place.

It was a miracle of advancement.

Not long ago Mr Cobb was predicting that they might have to amputate. Now the leg was as firm as a rock. No bandages. No elastic stocking.

No pain.

All this was incredible, but I think Andrew's words in his letter following his check-up one year after this trail-blazing operation summed it up in a nutshell:

> Dad, when I saw the latest X-rays I could hardly believe my eyes. Because there, in black and white, was hard evidence of bone growth! It was actually weaving its way into all the gaps, even filling up the gap between the bone and the prosthesis where Mr Cobb said he'd been unable to ground the prosthesis. It was amazing to see, since for the last thirteen years all I'd seen, year after year, was bone deterioration.
>
> Mr Cobb was really pleased, and if he'd had the chance I'm sure he would have broken into song! He had some photographs taken and said he was going to show me off – whatever that means! When I asked him if I could start playing golf again, he said by all means I could start swinging a club. But you know what? After thirteen years I'd be completely out of practice. I shall start on the practice tee. But, nah, whether I actually walk around a course again is doubtful.
> Yeah. I think I'd quite like to preserve my wonderful new bits of metal!

- 0 -

Sense at last, I thought when I read it, tears streaming down my face so much that I had to read it again.

I was so intrigued by what Andrew had told me about the bone growth that I wanted to know more about it. I had to find out everything I could. It was the most exciting news we'd had for a long time. Not since that fateful day all those years ago when Philip had told

296

us that Andrew might not have to lose his leg; not since the triumphant day when Mr Sweetnam saved his leg, had we heard such amazing news.

Andrew, with his eternal quest for wanting to know what was happening to his leg and often initiating events in true 'singing his own song' fashion, had already contacted Dr Blunn at the Biomedical Engineering Department at Stanmore, who jointly with Mr Cobb had been responsible for the original idea for the type of fixation method. Andrew gave me his number and as soon as I could I phoned him.

I introduced myself and said how fascinated I was and asked him how on earth this incredible bone growth had come about.

He told me that as an academic he very rarely got any form of personal feedback from patients and seemed very keen to talk to me and Andrew.

"Two different coatings are applied to the prosthesis," he explained. "One is a layer of Hydroxyapatite. This is a material which is naturally found in bone and is applied to the parts of the prosthesis that interface with the metal alloy. This increases the bone attachment to the implant to produce a more durable fixation. The other coating is titanium nitride. This is applied to the shaft of the implant and is a very hard layer. It prevents wear of the implant by soft tissue rubbing, and should reduce the tissue staining."

I swallowed hard. This was amazing. This to me was science fiction stuff. "Andrew will be very pleased about that," I said when I got my breath back. "And how long do you think this new prosthesis will last?" It would be too awful, I thought, if he had to have it all done again in a few years' time.

"Hopefully for Andrew's entire life," Dr Blunn replied.

Oh wow! I could hardly believe my ears. "That's fantastic! Does this mean he will never need to have another operation?"

"Hopefully, no - apart from the knee joint component which may need exchanging now and then because of problems associated with wear and tear. You see, the goal of Biomedical Engineering is to produce implants which last the patient's life-time and this is why we need to follow-up Andrew throughout his life. He is part of an on-going clinical trial for these implants."

"And when will the trials be complete?"

Dr Blunn laughed. "They never will be, really. Andrew and other patients in the trial are in the process of making medical history. But

297

there will always be room for improvement," he added.

I thought of Philip and Jo. If Philip had not intervened when he did, none of this would have been happening. There would have been no leg onto which to fit a prosthesis. Neither the original one, designed by Professor Scales and so miraculously fitted by Mr Sweetnam, nor this new marvel of Mr Cobb's and Dr Blunn's.

"Are these new prostheses successful so far?" I asked, not really wanting to hear the answer unless it was positive.

"So far there have been about twenty of these implants," he said. "Andrew was the seventh. Only one of the early ones failed but that's because we didn't get the design right. So yes, it's a pretty good success rate." Oh, the typical modesty of the man.

"Did Mr Cobb do them all?"

"He's done fifteen of them. He's the pioneer of this new surgery. He is one of the most innovative orthopaedic surgeons I know."

Speaking to Andrew the next day I was full of praise for Mr Cobb. "You're lucky to have such a wonderful doctor. You must think the world of him."

"I think he's marvellous, Mum. But then why wouldn't I?" He paused. "They've all been marvellous. Without Sir Rodney and Dr Jelliffe, I wouldn't even be here now."

I turned away to hide that insistent tear of mine. "Well, isn't it terrific that at last we can stop worrying about you losing your leg!"

"Mum!" he answered with amazement. "You of all people must have known that deep down I've always been sure I would never lose my leg!"

Chapter Thirty-one

The frogs are croaking. The crickets are chirping. The voices are all around me ...

I hold the body close. I sob. I scream. I try to coax the life back into it. I will it to breathe. I shout as loudly as I can:

Live! Live! Live!

I close my eyes and wait.

Suddenly the voices are fainter.

Now there's a buzzing in my ears.

Soon there is only the buzzing.

And now there is nothing but silence. I open my eyes.

Where have they all gone?

The moon has dipped low in the sky. It shines straight through the window now, catches me in its silver spotlight but still I do not look down.

I force my eyes upwards to the leaves that tremble on the ceiling. I must never look down at that blemished flesh again. I must close my eyes tightly, shut out the moonlight and the shadows and the body ...

But something is forcing my head down. An iron bar, pushing it down, down, down ...

No! Please don't make me look again.

Temptation overwhelms me. Sucks my eyelids apart. Drags my eyes open. A little at a time. Drags them towards the once perfect body I still clutch in my arms.

First it is only the light of the moon that I see.

Then —

What?

No! Impossible!

The body has gone!

The space between my eyelids widens. I see the dawn begin to break. The moon fades. Turns a milky white against the lightening grey of the sky, and stretching out in front of me I see a giant expanse of ice. Pale grey at first, but quickly turning to pinkish white, a blush of

299

coral on the horizon.

I skate towards it.

I see a blaze of orange. An explosion of flame as the sun bursts over the ice.

Faster and faster I skate towards it. It draws me like a magnet.

And then –

Oh no! It cannot be ...

Oh yes! It is!

Slowly, and very gently so that it will not disintegrate or mysteriously dissolve beneath my fingers and my eyes, I touch the body.

Gingerly I hold it at arms' length to get a better view – in case my eyes are deceiving me.

There are no gaping holes in this flesh.

No blood.

There are no imperfections in this flesh

No lacerations or shards of jagged bone to mar its beauty.

It is ... perfect.

I laugh.

I think.

Could it be a trick of the sun? Sent to mock me?

I wait and gaze. But still it looks perfect.

And then, in case it should suddenly vanish I crush it to my chest and run my hands over the cheeks the neck the chest the legs and Oh dear God, it is perfect again.

The sun shines down and I let my eyes feast on the wondrous eurhythmy of the rippling movement I see.

I must never let this moment go. I must hold on to it forever. For in all my life I will never see anything again so beautiful as this.

- 0 -

I never had the dream again.

Though sometimes, at the dead of night, when the frogs are croaking and the crickets are chirping and the moon casts its ethereal shadows on the stark white of the walls, I imagine I can see the glint of a knife blade, flashing ...

- 0 -

300

And what of Andrew's dreams?

He still dreams.
For what is life without dreams?

Postscript

Andrew won the Rodman Trophy for the second year running.

Shortly afterwards he was promoted to Flying Officer in the RAF Volunteer Reserve, Training Branch; and in addition to his job as an Air Traffic Controller at British Aerospace, Woodford, devoted all his spare time helping to run 391 (Wilmslow) Squadron Air Training Corps, instilling in the young cadets his passion for flying.

In 1999 he took up the post of Senior Air Traffic Control Officer at Royal Air Force, Wyton, thereby fulfilling his dream to work with the RAF. This challenging job entailed negotiating with the Civil Aviation Authority and the RAF in order to re-open the airfield after several years of closure and neglect.

"It's unbelievable," he said on his appointment. "Fifteen years ago, who'd have thought I'd be working with the Royal Air Force? It's a dream come true."

In 2004 he studied at City University London and in 2006 we attended his graduation in London, rejoicing in his success of being granted the degree of Master of Science in Air Transport Management.

Going from strength to strength, he moved to Brussels in 2006 where he took up a position working on European Single Sky policies at EUROCONTROL, focusing on safety.

Aviation Safety was fast becoming Andrew's major field of expertise, and in January 2011 he accepted a position as a member of the Airspace Safety Team at NATS – National Air Traffic Services Headquarters, located between Portsmouth and Southampton.

Throughout his Air Traffic career, Andrew has continued to serve as a member of the RAF Volunteer Reserve and was a founder of the RAF Air Cadet Junior Leaders' Course. He was also the Officer Commanding of Newmarket Squadron Air Training Corps, and was privileged to be able to help with Portsmouth Squadron during his time at NATS.

In addition he has, for the last eleven years, been invited to be one of the prestigious 'Follow-me' drivers at the annual Royal International Air Tattoo at RAF Fairford, where he has led the famous Red Arrows display team.

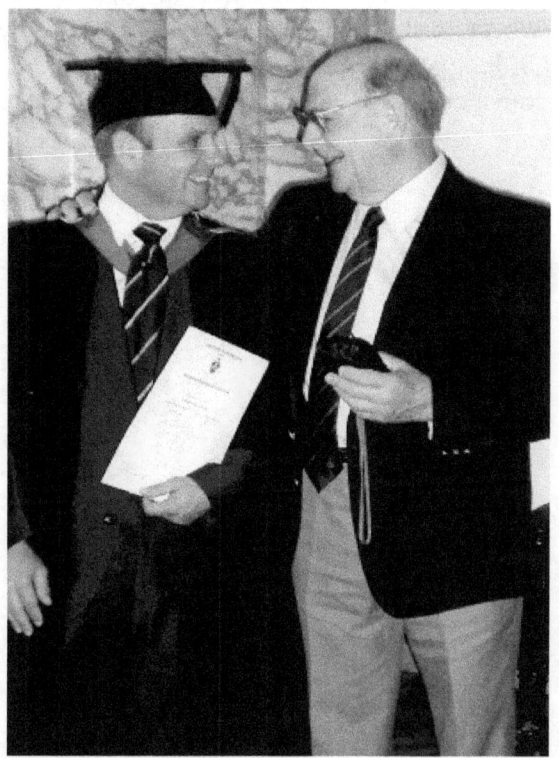

Congratulated by Dad at Graduation Ceremony in London

Always seeking new and more challenging ways to serve the aviation industry, especially in the all-important sphere of aviation safety, Andrew continues to make further major steps to pursue his career in Aviation Safety and is now a Registered Aviation Consultant with the British Association of Aviation Consultants.

- 0 -

Since the final major revision operation, Andrew has only had to have further surgery once to repair the prosthesis.

He still walks with a stick made by his father way back in 1985, lovingly whittled away from a fallen olive branch in our garden in a Menorcan Natural Park.

303

Very recently, after a new bout of pain necessitated a check-up by Professor Justin Cobb, the scans showed that more surgery is necessary. However, Justin has said "It's better they stay away from each other for as long as possible!"

Andrew is convinced that even then, we will still be able to count all ten of his toes.

Epilogue

It's a time of my life I wish I could forget but am unable to do so entirely. Luckily for me the brain has an uncanny way of blocking out the worst experiences, and it's really only after reading my mother's manuscript and the extracts from my diary that I'm reminded of what a nightmare it was. Not only for me but also for my parents, my family and my friends.

Although the events of 1984 only spanned a short period of my life, that short period still feels like a lifetime. I can still remember the horror of chemotherapy though I know that without it I wouldn't be here now. I can still remember the pain of the first operation to replace my knee and tibia, hoping I would never again have to endure such agony.

I can still remember the fear of losing my leg.

I had signed a consent form to an amputation and I was scared. Boys of eighteen are supposed to be tough but I was terrified. I knew that when I woke up from the operation I would have either two legs or one. I wouldn't know immediately. Grandpa, who had lost both his legs because of acute arteriosclerosis, had told me about the 'phantom limb'. About how the mind doesn't register the loss of a limb until quite some time after the event. About how one can actually feel it is still there, and feel the pain and even want to scratch an exact itchy spot on the non-existent limb and how the scratching actually relieves the itch. I knew this too from Tom's experience.

When I saw Dad's note on my pillow the sense of relief was overwhelming. 'I have counted your toes and there are ten!'

From that moment on I knew I no longer had cancer. I was on the road to recovery. I had my whole life in front of me and I was going to live every minute of it to the full. Surely my father could not have appreciated how much those few words on the back of his business card would mean to me. Words that somehow epitomised in my mind the love he had for me as a father.

As Dad has always said, "You know what they do to you in hospitals? Well, first they hurt you, but then they make you better."

I'd been hurt but I was going to get better. 'Why do I have to have more chemo? I don't have cancer anymore!' I was going to get well again, but it wasn't going to be easy.

Twenty-seven years later I am still incredibly well. I have my mother and father to thank, Philip and Jo, my family and my friends, and the ever supportive and dedicated team at The Middlesex Hospital (sadly no longer in existence) and the London Bone Tumour Clinic. Without them I could not, and would not have the quality of life I have today.

Someone once said to Grandpa Taylor, "How can you live like that without any legs?"

He replied, "Life is sweet."

And you know, he was so right. Despite the hardships one has to endure, there is always someone else out there in a worse position than you are; and I know that with the support I get from Mum and Dad, Sally, Rebecca and Alex, my amazing brothers – Colin and Peter – Philip and Jo, and many others – too many to mention but they know who they are – life will continue to be sweet.

I am so fortunate.

My life has been enriched by my experience.

If there is a target in my life now it is to tell people never to give up. To remember that life is sweet, no matter how turbulent the air, how steep the turns they must execute.

Mine has been a long flight, a bumpy flight, with sudden troughs of agony and soaring heights of ecstasy. The route was sometimes hazardous, sometimes enthralling, but it taught me many things –

How to be patient.

How to think more of other people's needs than my own.

How to give more than I receive.

How to savour every day as though it were my last.

I often think about my father and remember that magical number; and I count to ten ...